60 tips

fertility

Anne Dufour

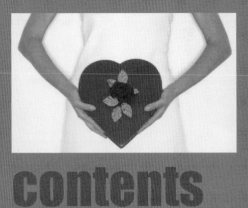

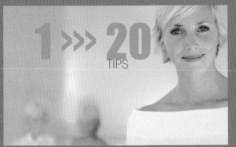

1 >>> 20 TIPS

contents

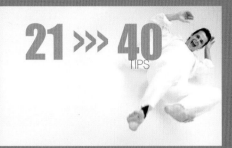

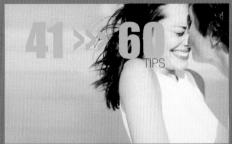

introduction

often there's not much wrong

A discourse on love

Have you been trying to conceive without any success for several months? Strictly medical reasons, such as hormonal imbalance, on either the female or the male side, can prevent pregnancy, and in such circumstances only the appropriate medical treatment will put the matter right. But in the great majority of cases there's plenty you can do personally to improve your fertility. The success rate for conception occuring during intercourse is only mediocre. This is not due to any fault in the 'basic materials' involved: female eggs are very efficient and well protected, while tens of millions of sperm are released during every intimate moment under the duvet, or elsewhere. A little love and passion should suffice to ensure that there are regular opportunities for one of the former to get to know one of the latter (not to mention opportunities for you to have a bit of fun while they do so). But returns are still limited: there is hardly a 25 per cent chance of a woman becoming pregnant during sexual intercourse, even if both partners are in the best of health.

Out of 100 couples having regular and complete sexual intercourse, about 25 will achieve pregnancy during the first menstrual cycle. Of the remaining 75, between 15 and 20 will succeed during the following month. The next month, a similar proportion (roughly 20 per cent) may expect to fall pregnant, and so on. So, by the end of a year, 16 per cent will not have conceived. By the end of the second year, 8 of the original 100 couples will still not have fallen pregnant. This unlucky 8 per cent will now usually be classed as having low fertility, for a variety of reasons. However, often these people simply need to adopt a healthier lifestyle in order to catch up with the rest.

Seeking medical assistance

Until now, couples who could not have children of their own were faced with a limited choice: adoption or childlessness. Now, though, physicians know much more about the various causes of infertility, and, where appropriate, they can prescribe assisted reproductive techniques (ART). Such courses of treatment have their merits and their limitations. The specialists always warn patients not to raise their hopes too high, and stress that the treatment will be long, difficult and often subject to side-effects. Before embarking upon treatment, you need to be aware that it's never straightforward. What's more, there's the possibility that your relationship itself might not be able to withstand such stress. Nevertheless, these medical procedures have obviously been a godsend for many. They have enabled thousands of couples to start a family, who probably never would have conceived in the conventional way, and ART is clearly the best option for all cases of subfertility caused by hormonal or organic problems. But in many other cases, the answer may be found elsewhere.

Men and women

In Europe, about 14 per cent of couples have trouble conceiving. The problem can be attributed to the man in 19 per cent of the cases and to the woman in between 40 and 50 per cent. In about 30 per cent, no cause for the infertility can be found. Female infertility often has a gynaecological origin, such as tubal problems or endometriosis, but it may be hormonal – for example, underactive thyroid or ovulatory problems. Male infertility is generally caused by often unknown factors which lead to a reduction in the number and effectiveness of the sperm.

Because there are so many unanswered questions about infertility, specialists have devoted a great deal of time and energy to studying the problem. They have considered our lifestyles, what we eat and the effects of pollutants, and have gone on to conduct tests, coordinate research and collect masses of information. The sum of this knowledge has been brought together in this book.

1 + 1 = 3

A baby is the product of the union of the genetic materials of its parents. Its conception and future health depend on these materials. Eating the most suitable food, leading a more healthy lifestyle, avoiding products with a toxic effect on the reproductive organs, and approaching the desired pregnancy calmly and sensibly all help to achieve conception itself and ensure that your baby starts life with the best possible chances of being healthy.

The 60 recommendations that follow are based upon the conclusions of many recent studies on the body's needs during the crucial time that precedes conception. All are easy to put into practice, although they may sometimes require some determination.

how to use this book

● ● ● FOR YOUR GUIDANCE

> A symbol at the bottom of each page will help you to identify the natural solutions available:

Herbal medicine, aromatherapy, homeopathy, Dr Bach's flower remedies – how natural medicine can help.

Simple exercises – preventing problems by strengthening your body.

Massage and manipulation – how they help to promote well-being.

Healthy eating – all you need to know about the contribution it makes.

Practical tips for your daily life – so that you can prevent instead of having to cure.

Psychology, relaxation, Zen – advice to help you be at peace with yourself and regain serenity.

> A complete programme that will solve all your health problems. Try it!

This book offers a made-to-measure programme, which will enable you to deal with your own particular problem. It is organized into four sections:

• **A questionnaire** to help you to assess the extent of your problem.
• **The first 20 tips are especially for women.**
• **The next 20 are more relevant to men.**
• **The final 20 concern both men and women.**

Case studies at the end of each section relate different people's experiences.

You can go through the book methodically, from Tip 1 to 60, putting each piece of advice into practice. Or you can follow those recommendations that seem particularly suited to your needs, habits and lifestyle. It's up to you!

are you sure you're doing all you can?

You've been to see your doctor. There doesn't seem to be anything medically wrong, and yet you are unable to conceive. If some of the statements below apply to you, perhaps they have some bearing on your infertility. Fortunately, you can do something about it!

	Him	Her	Both
You are hooked on dieting			
You were on the pill or used an IUD for a long time			
You have stomach problems (diarrhoea, vomiting)			
You have been pregnant within the last two years			
You are very overweight or very thin			
You smoke			
You drink alcohol			
You are a firefighter, a baker or spend all day driving			
You work in a laundry			
You don't eat a lot of fruit and vegetables			
You make love once a week or less			
You are older than 35			
You take drugs			
You are stressed and worried			
You are unsatisfied with your lifestyle			

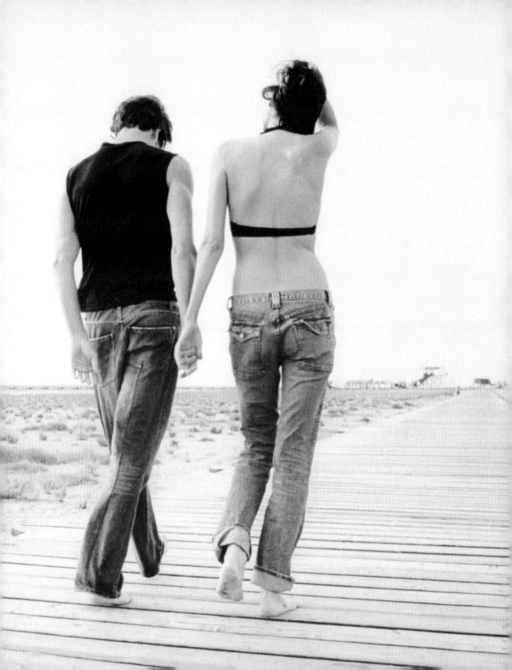

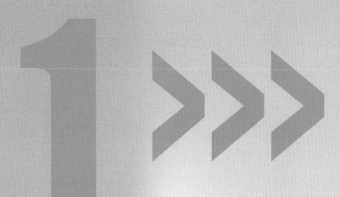

>> So you want to be a mum. You feel you are ready for parenthood and so is your partner.

>>>> You are in one of two situations: either you've been trying for some months and nothing has happened; or you want to plan for your pregnancy and prepare your body before it begins.

>>>>>> You've come to the right place! All budding mums (even those who have already had a child) ought to look through the following pages. They'll find all that we know today about the best ways of preparing for these very special nine months in the life of a woman and giving the baby the best possible start in life.

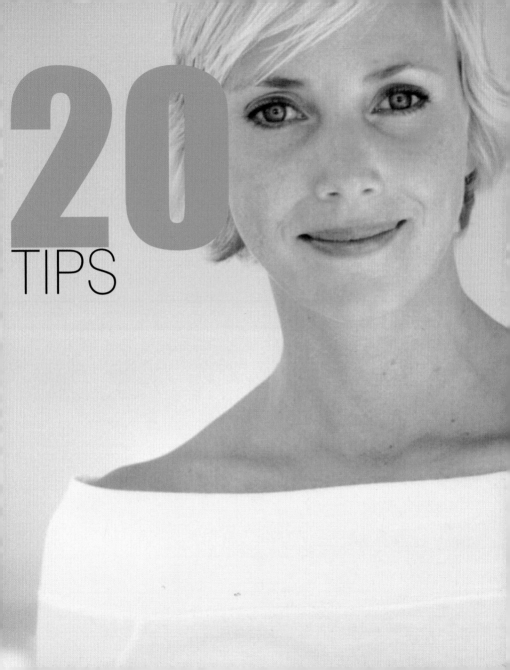

20
TIPS

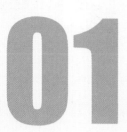

01

You need to take care of your body if you are going to conceive. This involves eating correctly, which means (good) proteins, (good) fats and (good) sugars at each of the three main meals.

eat better, eat well

The earlier, the better

It also means plenty of vitamins, minerals and beneficial nutrients. This may seem obvious, but the majority of women suffer from a lack of some of the nutrients they need at this time. Although you may have promised yourself you will improve your diet once you fall pregnant, it's just as important to do so beforehand. In fact, it's during the very first weeks of pregnancy that the cells of the foetus are most at risk from unsuitable eating.

● ● ● DID YOU KNOW?

> Researchers at the School of Public Health at Harvard (Boston, Mass.) have compiled a guide to the healthiest foods. They advocate the consumption of: unsaturated fats, particularly from vegetables and oily fish; fewer cereals and starchy foods; very little or no white rice, white bread, potatoes or pasta; very little delicatessen produce and red meat; far fewer dairy products (1 portion per day); much more fruit and fresh vegetables; more white meat and fish; a little red wine (rather than none); a daily dose of vitamin and mineral supplements.

Before, during and after

The first three weeks are therefore crucial if the foetus is to grow healthily, but the mother-to-be doesn't always know at that point that she is pregnant. Ideally, she should plan her pregnancy so she can build up her store of beneficial nutrients. This is particularly important in the case of women who smoke, the over-35s, those with dark skin and those who rarely expose themselves to sunlight. The same applies to inveterate dieters and those who were using an IUD or the pill.

Pregnant women should take folic acid as soon as they start to try for a baby and, because of contamination by heavy metals, consumption of certain sea fish, including tuna, swordfish and mackerel, should be restricted to once or twice a month.

> In the UK, especially to prevent spina bifida and hydrocephalus (neural-tube defects), the Department of Health advises women to take 400mcg of folic acid daily, from when they first start trying for a baby until the 13th week of pregnancy. (See Tip 9 for more information about folic acid.)

KEY FACTS

* Eat enough, but not too much!

* Eat more fruit and vegetables, and less meat and dairy products.

* Take folic acid as soon as you try for a baby.

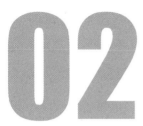

02

put on a
little weight...

One woman in three is convinced she's overweight when she's not. One in two is concerned about her figure. One in five is permanently on a diet. This irrational search for an 'ideal' slim figure can be a direct cause of infertility.

Everything slows down

The obsession with slimness at all costs can blight your life for years, and you might pay dearly for each drastic diet when you want to start a family. Given that not eating enough food for just four days is enough to disturb our delicate hormonal balance, it is easy to imagine the potential damage caused by years of dieting. Everything slows down in women who diet continually, including the production of sex hormones. The

● ● ● D I D   Y O U   K N O W ?

> Besides not providing the body with all the macronutrients (proteins, sugars and fats) it needs to function, eating too little deprives us of necessary micronutrients (see right).

> 70 per cent of women lack folic acid (vitamin B9); 66 per cent lack iron; 40 per cent lack magnesium; and nearly 80 per cent lack zinc.

body goes into survival mode: not knowing if it's going to get enough calories each day to sustain itself, it cannot allow itself to conceive a baby, and eventually ovulation fails and periods stop. You don't have to have anorexia nervosa for this to happen, and sometimes a weight gain of as little as 3–4kg (half a stone/7lb) will be enough to trigger ovulation again.

Femininity = fertility

Most women hate having chubby buttocks and thighs, yet these represent reserves of energy vital in pregnancy. What's more, men rarely make any objection to such signs of femininity. So why do we insist on getting rid of what so obviously pleases our partners? You can also find yourself in this situation – too much muscle and not enough fat – if you do a lot of intense physical exercise. When trying for a baby, being underweight is more of a disadvantage than being overweight.

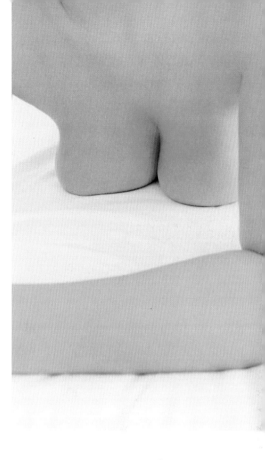

> All of these substances play a vital part in the process of reproduction. Some doctors prescribe nutritional supplements of these 'fashion victims' as a matter of course.

KEY FACTS

* Being too thin makes it more likely that you'll be infertile.

* Merely putting on a little weight can help a woman to conceive.

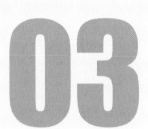

03

Being overweight, particularly if you are classed as obese, can hinder the reproductive process from ovulation onwards. What's more, those superfluous kilos increase the risk of complications during pregnancy.

... or lose some!

Anorexia, bulimia, the consequences are the same

Not only anorexia and bulimia, but all eating disorders, particularly those that involve going from one extreme of food intake to the other, disturb ovulation. Most doctors agree that there is a close link between gynaecology and weight, and this is particularly true of ovulation problems. Although it may better to be

● ● ●   D I D   Y O U   K N O W ?

> If you are overweight and trying to become pregnant, you need to lose weight for the sake of your own and your baby's health. Diet sensibly and exercise for 20 mins most days.
> Obese women who are pregnant are considerably more likely to suffer from high blood pressure and diabetes, to need a

Caesarean section and even to die.
> Overweight women are more liable to suffer from illnesses often associated with pregnancy, such as urinary infections and circulation problems.
> The baby runs a greater risk of death if the mother is obese.

too fat rather than too thin if you want to conceive, it's undeniably best of all to be within the normal weight range.

Fats, the source of hormones

Clearly, obesity doesn't necessarily lead to infertility, because many extremely overweight women have children. However, the more a woman is over-weight, the greater the risk of infertility. In addition, excessive weight hinders infertility treatments. Once again, it's all a matter of hormones, as the amount of fat in the body has a great bearing on the levels of several hormones. Obesity is associated with the development of polycystic ovaries and inefficient ovula-tion by a mechanism involving the over-production of insulin. This contributes to a woman being three times more likely to have problems ovulating if she is very overweight. In most cases, however, obese women who make the effort to lose a few kilos return to perfectly nor-mal monthly cycles once they have done so. Exercise, even without major weight loss, also helps normalize insulin metabolism and improves ovulation.

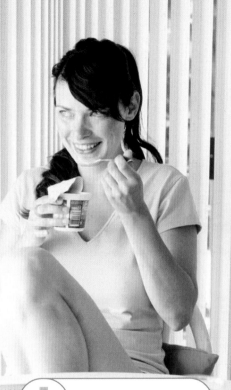

KEY FACTS

* Being overweight disturbs the monthly cycle and can reduce fertility.

* But don't undertake drastic diets that deprive you of sufficient nourishment.

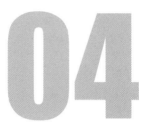

Stress is perhaps the biggest killer in the Western world. And its power to harm even extends to preventing you from having children. Make getting rid of it one of your priorities.

don't let stress get you down

The dangers of stress

Stress always has an effect on the body. Sometimes we are aware of its physical symptoms (stomach aches, heavy sweating and so on), but it also causes much more serious and, significantly, more permanent damage. Often, it has an insidious effect on our internal organs, including the reproductive system.

● ● ● DID YOU KNOW?

> Stress isn't necessarily harmful. Without it, our cavemen ancestors would not have survived. Stress is stimulating: it drives us on, leads us to change our job or partner should we be unhappy and generally adds spice to our lives. Things would be very dull without it!

> However, daily, repetitive stress causes a great deal of harm. To conceive a child, even to want one in the first place, you need to feel confident and relaxed. So try to de-stress and make a little space for the new addition to your family.

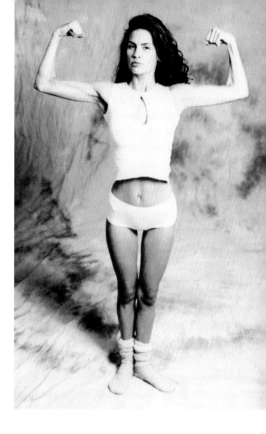

Day after day

Even ordinary, day-to-day stress can have a profound effect on fertility by contributing to the cessation of ovulation. Everyday examples include periods stopping when a woman travels or when young women leave home for the first time to go to university. Not only can stress affect the number of eggs fertilized, but also the birth weight of babies, particularly in the case of multiple pregnancies. You need to avoid feeling stressed at all times. Have a rest, take it easy, do something just for yourself, enjoy a massage, avoid noise, try to stay calm, take some exercise (non-contact martial arts are particularly recommended). Above all, reserve some time in your busy schedule just for yourself. And don't forget that our nerve cells need nourishment, too. Well-balanced meals generally provide a good basis for relaxation.

KEY FACTS

* Too much stress can even reduce your desire to have a child.

* Set some time aside in your busy schedule for relaxation.

* Forget your worries; think of something else.

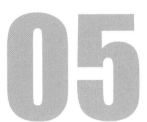

05

get your timing right

One in five couples has difficulty conceiving a child, even though everything is 'working well'. It could be that they are just not making love at the right time.

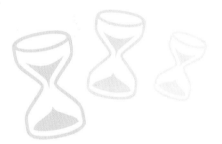

Opening the window

The 'window of fertility' refers to the period of time when the cervical mucus 'accepts' the sperm. For the rest of the month, it is too acidic and destroys the sperm. To find out if you are in this 'window', insert one or two fingers into your vagina and collect the mucus that is in contact with the neck of the uterus, or cervix. Just after a monthly period, there's hardly any mucus at all; later, it

●●● D I D   Y O U   K N O W ?

> In theory, a woman can only conceive on certain days of the month. Ovulation occurs about two weeks before a period, so the 14th day of a regular 28-day cycle should be the most fertile. As sperm can live for around four days in the female genital tract, four days either side of day 14 should also be

fertile. Therefore the most likely time for conception is between the 10th and 17th days of a monthly cycle. (NB the first day of the monthly cycle corresponds to the first day of a period.)

> In reality, however, only 30 per cent of women are this regular. For the

becomes thick and sticky. Approaching ovulation, it becomes clear and flows more freely and will stretch between two fingers, which is a good pointer. During this (brief) period, the mucus will extend a warm welcome to the sperm.

All women are different

Be careful not to confuse cervical mucus with ordinary vaginal discharge. There is a simple way to tell them apart. After taking a sample of the secretion, put your finger in a glass of water. If the mucus dissolves, it is vaginal discharge; if it does not, it is cervical mucus. The result, however, can be distorted by infection, sexual excitement, recent sexual intercourse (sperm will be mingled with the secretion) or the presence of a lubricant. Nevertheless, with a little care and attention to detail, it is easy to learn when your 'window of fertility' occurs, particularly if your monthly cycle is regular.

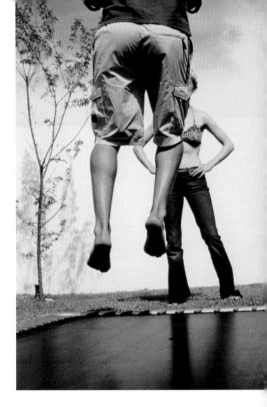

rest, the fertile period changes every month.
> This 'window of fertility' can prove elusive, and demanding your partner performs by the calendar can turn intercourse into a chore. Concentrate on having a good time in bed and making love two or three times each week, without ever checking the date!

KEY FACTS

* The 14th day of the cycle is theoretically the most fertile.

* But there are many factors that can disturb the monthly cycle.

* Learn to understand when your body is at its most fertile, but don't let it dictate your love life.

You can increase your intake of vitamins and minerals by changing your cooking methods. Choose gentler methods, so that your food remains nutritious but loses none of its flavour.

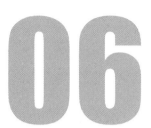

06

change the way you cook

Choosing and preparing

Choosing food that contains plenty of vitamins is good. Cooking it correctly is even better. Remember that vitamins are sensitive to both heat and light, while minerals are leached out of food by water. To get the full benefit of the nutrients in fruit and vegetables, store them in a dark, cool place and use gentle cooking methods – and not too much water. Raw vegetables and salad make a good

● ● ● DID YOU KNOW?

> The best cooking methods for preserving vitamins in food are steaming and braising.
> Steaming is definitely the simpler method, but braising is better for all foods that generate water and produce juices.

> A golden rule when steam cooking is to always bring the water to the boil before putting the food into the basket.

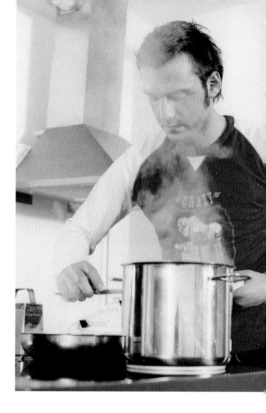

starter, as long as you go easy on the vinaigrette. Eat at least two pieces of raw fruit per day: this is a good way of stocking up on vitamin C and the roughage needed to avoid constipation.

Losing minerals

Heat improves flavour, helps in the absorption of nutrients and removes certain toxins. Cooking is a kind of 'pre-digestion' that reduces the workload of the stomach and frees vital energy, which can then be put to other uses. But when it's done incorrectly, it causes minerals to be lost into the water, destroys vitamins and even creates carcinogenic substances (especially during grilling and frying).

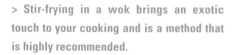

> Stir-frying in a wok brings an exotic touch to your cooking and is a method that is highly recommended.

07 take your temperature

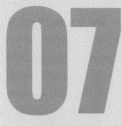

Although superseded in clinics by more sophisticated techniques, some people use their temperature curve to help predict ovulation.

> Your temperature curve records the development of your whole cycle. It can help you predict ovulation and may also provide an early indication of a pregnancy.

> There are two phases in the course of the monthly cycle: a phase of 'low' temperatures before ovulation and a phase of 'high' ones after. If conception has not taken place, the temperature falls again and the period occurs, followed by the beginning of a new cycle.

A strict routine

Your body temperature curve varies in accordance with your hormonal clock. Ovulation, especially, causes an increase in temperature within the monthly cycle. Recording the curve enables any disorder in the cycle to be detected. You will need to use a special thermometer that enables you to read body temperature very accurately, as the variations are quite small. When correctly interpreted, the temperature curve provides valuable information about ovulation, but you will need to keep a record of the curve for at least three months. All you need to do is take your temperature every morning before you get up, keep a note of it on paper and plot it on graph paper. It doesn't matter where you take your temperature (mouth, vagina, rectum or under the arm), provided that you keep to the same place, use the same thermometer and do it at the same time every day.

Temperature variations

Make sure your graph is big enough to allow the temperature variations between 36° and 37°C (96.8° and 98.6°F) to be clearly seen. A word of warning: the results are distorted if you work at night, are very stressed, have drunk alcohol the evening before, are suffering from a fever, or if you have recently undergone a course of hormonal treatment (all treatments involving a base of oestrogens or progestogen, including the pill).

> You will need to use a basal body thermometer that enables you to read temperature very accurately, as the variations are quite small. These special thermometers often come with a standardized chart on which to record your temperature readings.

KEY FACTS

* The temperature curve can help predict ovulation.

* You need to keep a record of the temperature curve for at least three months.

08

think about contraception

Obviously, if you want to have a baby, you must stop using all forms of contraception, but it might also be an idea to change to a different method in the three months *before* you want conception to occur.

Long live the condom!

Of course, the method of contraception that suits you best ultimately depends on your personal preferences and lifestyle. However, some methods are more suitable than others for those who wish to start a family in the near future. Perhaps the best in this respect are condoms (both female and male) used in conjunction with spermicides. The IUD, or coil, unfortunately, often causes heavy

● ● ● DID YOU KNOW?

> The time taken to regain fertility after the use of a contraceptive varies.

> For women aged over 30 who have been on the combined oral contraceptive pill, it can take from ten days to several months.

periods and could thereby lead to iron deficiency, but once it is removed fertility returns promptly.

The pill and other methods of birth control

Taking the pill does not usually make it more difficult to conceive later; indeed, some women conceive after forgetting to take it on just a few occasions. But, after coming off the pill, you should wait before trying to conceive until after your first period. This makes it easier for doctors to date the pregnancy should one occur. In contrast, if you use the progesterone injection form of birth control, when you cease this method your periods may be slow to return. It is, of course, most difficult to restore fertility after a vasectomy or the tying of the Fallopian tubes.

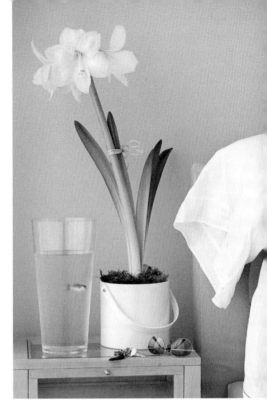

> With the progestogen-only pill, you may conceive again twelve hours after you stop taking it!

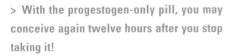

KEY FACTS

* Your fertility can depend on the method of contraception you have been using.

* Condoms and spermicides are good contraceptives to use in the three months leading up to the desired time of conception.

09

folic acid is a must!

Folic acid (vitamin B9) is essential for fertility and conception, and for the mother-to-be and baby. It is particularly vital just before a child is conceived and in the days immediately afterwards.

An indispensable vitamin

Folic acid has a crucial role to play in everything that affects DNA and genetic information. This essential vitamin increases female fertility and, in addition, helps to prevent the malformation of the neural tube in the foetus. Should this malformation occur, the baby would be exposed to a very serious condition: spina bifida. Folic acid begins this vital protection during the first weeks of

● ● ● DID YOU KNOW?

> One of the causes of male infertility is 'round cells syndrome', characterized by the presence of round (and therefore malformed) sperm. Folic acid supplements have produced good results among affected men.
> This vitamin (which is almost totally without side-effects for women of child-bearing age) protects against many other illnesses, especially cardiac disorders.
> In spite of these benefits, it is first and foremost known as a 'woman's vitamin'.
> Folic acid occurs naturally in a range of foods, including baker's

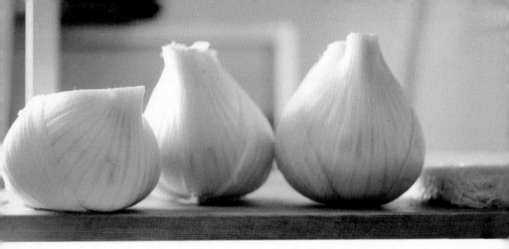

pregnancy, before the mother may even be aware that she is pregnant, so it is essential that the course of supplements is started before conception.

An essential supplement

For a variety of reasons, most women don't get enough folic acid from their diet alone: the body can only store the vitamin for three months, and it is easily destroyed during cooking. The mother-to-be should therefore 'stock up' on folic acid by taking it in the form of a supplement before she plans to conceive. She should then continue to take the supplement throughout the period of conception until 13 weeks into her pregnancy. The recommended dose to prevent spina bifida is 400mcg per day, but if there is a history of the condition in your family, consult your doctor who may prescribe a higher dosage.

yeast, wheatgerm, wholegrain wheat, spinach, egg yolk, calf's liver, fennel, cabbages, green beans and lettuces.
> It is also routinely added to common foodstuffs, such as flour, in parts of the Developing World because its health benefits are so pronounced.

KEY FACTS

* Folic acid is indispensable for pregnant women.

* Folic acid supplements are available from pharmacies.

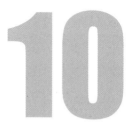

10

don't forget vitamin B12...

Every vitamin, mineral and trace element has its part to play, but some nutrients are particularly important during pregnancy. Vitamin B12 is one of the most crucial.

Vegans, take care!

In the West, few people suffer from B12 deficiency, because of the high consumption of meat. Vegetarians who consume eggs and dairy products are also not at risk. But vegans, who consume no products of animal origin whatsoever, may well suffer from the condition, because this vitamin is not found in plants. Strict vegans have just two, insignificant sources of B12 – yeast and bacteria – in

● ● ● D I D   Y O U   K N O W ?

> Tiredness and breathlessness are two conditions that could be early signs of a lack of B12, but there are many others: loss of appetite, anaemia, pins and needles (indicating damage to the nervous system), numbness and weakness in the legs.

> Other symptoms may include poor memory, depression, irritability and mood disturbances.
> B12 is needed to produce an adequate amount of healthy red blood cells in the bone marrow.

their diet. However, because the body is able to store B12 for up to three years, people whose diet is deficient in this might feel fine for some time, not realizing that they are exhausting their stocks. If you are a vegan, it is therefore advisable to take supplements of B12. You should also note that if you drink a lot of alcohol, it's likely that you will suffer from a shortage of other B group vitamins, especially thiamine (B1) and folic acid.

'Photocopying' DNA

Like folic acid, B12 plays a key part in cellular reproduction. By means of a complex process, it 'photocopies' DNA. In addition, B12 is necessary for the production of red blood cells, and it is vital for healthy nerve cells because it produces myelin, the white sheath that surrounds nerve fibres.

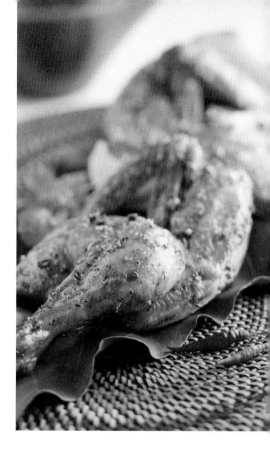

> B12 is found in abundance in shellfish, cow's liver, chicken, fish and eggs.

KEY FACTS

* Vitamin B12 is indispensable during pregnancy.

* Supplements, available over the counter from your pharmacy, can improve your fertility.

11

As well as folic acid, B12 and the minerals zinc and magnesium, you must make sure you get enough vitamin B6.

... and pyridoxine is vital, too

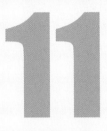

An important double act

Pyridoxine (B6) and magnesium are like Laurel and Hardy: there's no point having one without the other. If your body lacks B6, it cannot assimilate magnesium properly (see Tip 14). You may get enough of the mineral through a healthy diet, but your body will be unable to retain and use it. Pyridoxine also plays a key role in the metabolism of many amino acids, the building blocks of proteins, and it has

●●● DID YOU KNOW?

> Fluctuations in the level of oestrogen in the menstrual cycle are associated with mood changes, and the fall in oestrogen level just before the period may trigger the irritability and sensitivity known as pre-menstrual tension.

> Doctors believe that lack of pyridoxine is largely to blame for the starving sensation that affects many women during the pre-menstrual period, even though it's not yet known precisely why this occurs.

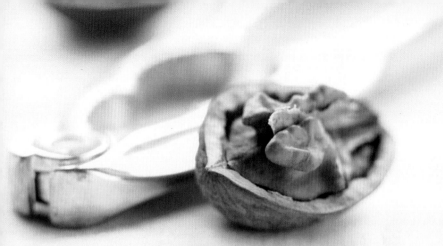

been used to treat pre-menstrual stress, but never exceed the recommended dose as damage to peripheral nerves can occur at high dosage.

The 'anti-stress' vitamin

Although a review of studies concluded that there was no definitive proof that vitamin B6 had an effect on the symptoms of PMS, many healthcare providers and their patients reported an improvement after using the vitamin. How well you respond to vitamin B6 may vary from person to person, so talk to your doctor about whether it is appropriate and safe for you. In addition to other B complex vitamins, pyridoxine is considered an 'anti-stress' vitamin as it is thought to enhance the body's immune system and improve its ability to combat stress. A recent review of scientific studies concluded that B6 may also help reduce the severity of nausea in early pregnancy.

> Fish, wheatgerm cereals, green vegetables, fruit, brewer's yeast and walnuts are all good sources of vitamin B6.

KEY FACTS

∗ Vitamin B6 allows the body to assimilate magnesium.

∗ It may be necessary to take supplements, which are widely available.

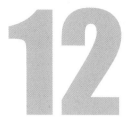

12 invest in a predictor kit

If you are finding it difficult to work out when your fertile period is, an ovulation predictor kit may be useful.

Safe and easy to use: Ovulation is triggered by the luteinizing hormone (LH), produced in the pituitary gland. To find out exactly when you are ovulating, buy a predictor kit, which will detect when you have the most LH in your urine. The peak occurs between 24 and 48 hours before ovulation. Ideally, carry out the test during your first urination of the day.

Using the kit: A kit usually consists of five test strips. It's easy to interpret the result: if the strip becomes strongly coloured, it indicates you are at the point in the cycle when you are most likely to fall pregnant. In your most fertile week, use a test strip each morning to calculate the best days. If your monthly cycle is regular, carry out the test 17 days before your period and in the days after. If not, it's best to test your urine over a longer period of time. However, try not to become a slave to the results. The kit might indicate that you are extremely fertile, but it doesn't guarantee that you will conceive that day. Equally, if the result is less encouraging, don't let that put you off trying for a baby if you and your partner are in the mood. These kits are meant to assist, not dictate to you.

● ● ● D I D Y O U K N O W ?

> During most of the menstrual cycle, only a small quantity of LH is secreted. In the middle of the cycle, the amount increases rapidly.
> The 'LH peak' sets off ovulation during the next 24 to 48 hours, the period in which conception is most likely to occur.

K E Y F A C T S

* An ovulation kit enables you to predict your most fertile period with accuracy. Use it to help you in your quest for a baby, but don't become a slave to it.

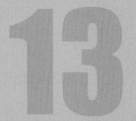

13 plant remedies can help

Traditional remedies are still being used today to stimulate the ovaries and to enhance fertility.

The benefits of herbal remedies: To boost fertility, Western herbal medicine above all advocates chastetree, which acts upon the pituitary gland and stimulates the hormones that trigger ovulation. Helionas (unicorn) root also stimulates the ovaries, while wild yam is used to regulate female hormones and improve the condition of the reproductive organs. However, don't embark on a course of herbal treatment by yourself on the grounds that 'it's natural so it can't do any harm'. Always consult a specialist.

Yin and yang: Chinese medicine considers infertility to be a 'disharmony' brought about by 'wet heat' and an imbalance between the yin and the yang. Practitioners prescribe hormonal tonics and plants that regulate the body's energies, such as ginseng and Chinese archangel. But these two plants should never be taken during pregnancy.

● ● ● DID YOU KNOW?

> Ayurvedic medicine utilizes plants to combat infertility. Shatavari root is reputed to be the most effective.

> Garlic, asparagus, onion, liquorice and fenugreek all stimulate the reproductive organs. Liquorice and fenugreek should not be taken when pregnant.

KEY FACTS

* Certain plants stimulate the hormonal system.

* Consult specialist practitioners. Do not try to treat yourself, as certain herbal remedies can be harmful, especially during pregnancy.

It's well known that magnesium is good for the nerves, especially if you are prone to muscle spasms. You also need plenty of it if you want to conceive.

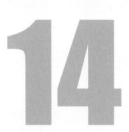

14

get plenty of magnesium

Stress and conception

Some doctors believe that magnesium deficiency is a major cause of non-organic infertility. In one trial, when infertile women with a low magnesium level took supplements, their fertility rate improved by 75 per cent. And those among the 25 per cent who didn't respond to the magnesium by itself, responded positively if it was combined with antioxidant supplements. Stress

● ● ● D I D Y O U K N O W ?

> In the 19th century, a French neurologist named Charcot called feminine muscle spasms 'hysteria (of the uterus)'.

> He thought this phenomenon resulted from stress caused by the 'terrible economic status' of women, from which there was no escape at the time.

reduces the body's ability to retain magnesium in the cells, which need to be repaired with the help of antioxidants.

Men can be affected, too

Although women may be more prone to hormonal deficiencies, men are not spared entirely. Stress drives magnesium from everyone's cells, and it is then excreted in the urine. The more stressed you are, the more magnesium you lose.

The best sources of the mineral are found in shellfish (especially whelks), cocoa powder, dried fruit, nuts, dates, spinach, chard (a variety of beet), green beans and cereals. Some brands of mineral water boast of very high levels of magnesium, too.

> He also blamed magnesium deficiency for muscular contractions. The uterus, like all muscles, he argued, could become tense and would contract as a result of stress.

KEY FACTS

* A healthy diet provides just about enough magnesium.

* You can supplement your intake of magnesium easily by drinking certain types of mineral water.

15 alternative therapies

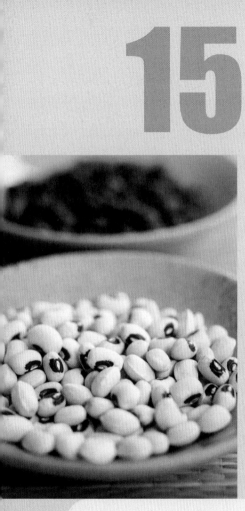

Alternative therapies can also play a part in helping to improve fertility. The benefits they bring are generally linked to helping reduce tension and stress and to paying attention to diet, in order to ensure that both partners are healthy and relaxed.

months before conception. It also stresses the importance of good health and gives nutritional advice.

> Traditional Chinese Medicine (TCM): this form of medicine makes use of a combination of acupuncture (see Tip 17) and herbal medicine, with the aim of increasing sperm mobility,

Autogenic training

Devised by Johannes Schultz in the 1920s, autogenic training is a form of relaxation therapy in which you use your mind to relax and reduce tension in the body. It consists of a series of six exercises that are carried out progressively. During each exercise, you concentrate upon a specific phrase in order to gain awareness of your body. The aim is to gain control of your breathing, heartbeat, your inner organs and your mind so that you can become totally relaxed at any time. By focussing on relaxing phrases and images, it teaches you to respond positively to verbal and visual cues.

As with most forms of alternative therapy, autogenic training should only be practised under the guidance of an approved practitioner It could be dangerous used incorrectly, or in the wrong circumstances. It could cause emotional problems and should not be used by people with mental disorders, or those with certain medical conditions, such as diabetes, heart conditions, glaucoma or high or low blood pressure. Consult your doctor before trying this therapy.

Aromatherapy

In this popular form of therapy, essential oils are extracted from plants and are used in different ways (vaporisation, massage, bathing) to help reduce tension. It is also thought that they may help to regulate women's fertility cycles. A qualified therapist must always be consulted because some essential oils must not be used during pregnancy.

KEY FACTS

* Don't confuse autogenic training with auto-suggestion. The latter is a form of self-hypnosis that uses meditation and the repetition of positive words or phrases to enhance well-being and help alleviate physical pain.

stimulating ovulation and increasing blood flow to the uterus. It also gives nutritional advice.

> Naturopathy: this comprises a range of natural therapies and healing techniques to help the body to heal itself.

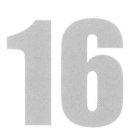

16

After childbirth, it may take some time for you to conceive again. And it could take even longer if you are breastfeeding your baby. This is all completely natural: your body needs to rest before another pregnancy.

be patient before trying again

A three-month wait ... at least

Pregnancy exhausts the body, particularly if you've had twins. It would be convenient if nature guaranteed you a rest so your body had a chance to replenish its stocks of nutrients before you could conceive again. And, to some extent, it does, through one of the side-effects of breast-feeding. But women who choose not to breastfeed must be aware that they could have their first period just six weeks after

● ● ● DID YOU KNOW?

> To give your body time to recover after childbirth, you should begin to use contraception immediately. Especially if you are using formula, it is possible to become pregnant again very quickly.

> Even if you wish to have another child as soon as possible, you should use contraception for several months at the very least to ensure that your body is in a good condition when the new embryo is created.

giving birth, and could therefore have two babies in under a year. Be careful: don't wait for your first period before using contraception as you will, of course, have ovulated two weeks prior to this.

It's all due to those hormones

If you are breastfeeding conception is inhibited, so it is sometimes considered an effective, natural method of contraception. You should, however, never rely upon it indefinitely: over the years, many women have conceived while breastfeeding. Prolactin, the hormone responsible for lactation, exerts its contraceptive effect by interfering with other pituitary hormones that stimulate the ovaries and by preventing ovulation and menstruation. This effect wears off over time and as the baby is weaned, but a mother with an infant under six months old is unlikely to conceive, provided she is exclusively breastfeeding and not menstruating.

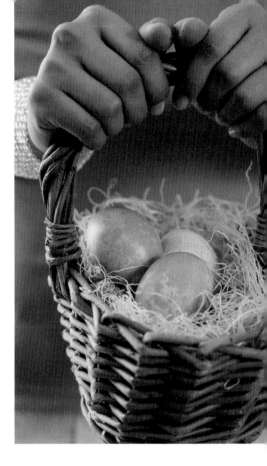

> If you have had a Caesarean section, you must allow time for the scar on the womb to heal before becoming pregnant again, and consult your doctor about how long to wait.
> Ideally, you should wait for a minimum of two years before becoming pregnant again.

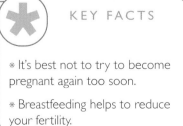

KEY FACTS

* It's best not to try to become pregnant again too soon.

* Breastfeeding helps to reduce your fertility.

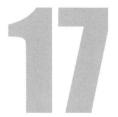

try acupuncture

Acupuncture can improve the success rate of in vitro fertilization. So why not natural fertilization, too?

Breathe in: A study carried out in Germany has shown that women having IVF treatment combined with acupuncture sessions have increased their chances of conception by 50 per cent, and have reduced the time they have to wait before it takes place. Although it is not yet known why this happens, there is good reason to believe that acupuncture generally improves fertility, even for women who have not had recourse to ART.

A relaxed uterus: In the German study, scientists separated 160 women into two groups: 80 had the conventional IVF treatment, while the other 80 benefited from an acupuncture session before and after the transfer of the embryo into the uterus. In this instance, needles were placed at points that were supposed to relax the uterus, but an acupuncturist may also stimulate certain points in order to improve hormonal balance.

● ● ● D I D Y O U K N O W ?

> Acupuncture is particularly suitable for treating minor problems that contribute to infertility. Its basic principle is that problems occur when the vital energy which circulates through the body, the qi, is impeded. It is now acknowledged as a credible form of treatment and is recommended by the WHO for a number of illnesses.

KEY FACTS

∗ Acupuncture can help to increase fertility.

∗ By restoring the flow of energy, the acupuncturist relieves the effects of 'blockages'.

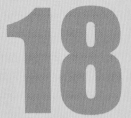

18 exercise your pelvic floor

It's a good idea to improve the condition of your pelvic floor. Even if toning it up won't directly increase your fertility, a little exercise won't do it any harm.

Breathe in: If you regularly exercise your pelvic floor muscles, you'll be able to detect changes in your secretions of cervical mucus. This will help identify the days when you are most likely to conceive, without needing to explore your private parts with your fingers. When you contract the muscles in your pelvic floor, you'll feel the moistness of your mucous membranes. Outside the period of fertility, this area seems dry and the labia are more difficult to separate.

How to do it: As often as you can during the day, tightly contract these muscles as if you were stopping yourself from going to the toilet. While waiting for the bus, walking down the street or sitting at your computer, contract them for a few seconds, relax them and then contract them again. When you are on the toilet, deliberately stop the flow of urine for a few seconds before continuing.

KEY FACTS

∗ The muscles of the pelvic floor need to be kept strong.

∗ They can help you to identify the days when you are most likely to conceive.

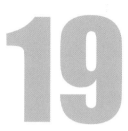

19

get just the right amount of iron

In the nineteenth century it was commonly assumed that women were generally deficient in iron. The combination of repeated pregnancies, miscarriage, heavy bleeding from disorders such as fibroids and poor diet made this a fairly safe assumption, and iron supplements were routinely prescribed.

An iron constitution

Nowadays, only pregnant women with demonstrated anaemia are offered iron supplements. If the slightest effort makes you breathless and you are always tired and irritable, finding it hard to sleep, you could be suffering from iron deficiency. Other signs are a pallid complexion and a raised heart rate. An adequate amount of this mineral is vital if our body and mind are to function well. Anaemia (a reduction in the number of red blood cells) may

● ● ● DID YOU KNOW?

> Iron is essential if you are planning a baby. A pregnant woman needs to double her intake to provide for the new baby. Iron is important for the tissues, the placenta and, of course, for the development of the embryo.
> A deficiency in iron makes you feel permanently tired and somewhat irritable, but a major shortage leaves you vulnerable to much more serious problems.
> But don't panic! Nature takes care of the situation: the body assimilates iron more efficiently during pregnancy than it does at other times.

affect 'only' 5 per cent of women in the Western world, but many more could suffer from iron deficiency. Since iron carries oxygen from the lungs to the muscles and all over the body, a shortage affects all aspects of health, including fertility.

From deficit to serious shortage

Each case needs to be examined individually, but it is known that IUDs and frequent pregnancies increase the risk of iron deficiency in women. The underlying cause of the deficiency could be inadequate intake (through poor diet) or excessive loss (through menstrual bleeding and bleeding caused by illnesses). Women who have heavy and/or long periods, those who have been pregnant in the last two years and those who are on a continuous diet are most prone to iron deficiency.

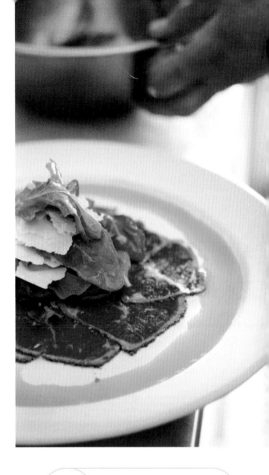

> Foods rich in iron are black pudding, red meat, liver, eggs, cocoa, lentils and parsley. and standard vitamin supplements with the recommended daily amount of iron are safe to take.

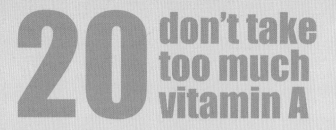

20 don't take too much vitamin A

Vitamin A is necessary for general health and fertility. But don't take too much of it, and be aware of the difference between the harmless kind and the kind that can cause problems.

Pride of place to beta-carotene: It's dangerous to think that vitamins are always good for you. Vitamin A, for example, is a tricky customer that can do you serious harm. On the plus side, there is no danger of consuming too much of the kind of vitamin A that is also known as beta-carotene or pro-vitamin A. This is found in fruit and vegetables, along with other vitamins and beneficial nutrients. It is metabolized in the body, but only on demand, and any excess is eliminated naturally.

Beware of calf's liver: On the other hand, the type of vitamin A that is found in animal products, also known as retinol, can pose problems for pregnant women: it can cause foetal deformities. So, if you like calf's liver enough to eat it every week, you'll have to deprive yourself until after you've given birth.

● ● ● DID YOU KNOW?

> Women who take the contraceptive pill may experience reduced levels of beta-carotene.

> They should double their intake of foods that are rich in beta-carotene: red peppers, paprika, carrots, apricots, spinach, watermelons, mangoes and lettuce.

> The main animal sources of vitamin A are cod liver oil, (calf's) liver, margarine, butter, eggs, fatty cheeses and full-cream milk.

KEY FACTS

* Eat more fresh fruit.

* Increase your daily intake of vegetables.

case study

« It's better now, my weight is back to normal, but you should have seen me before! Fred and I had made up our minds we wanted a baby. Although I'd never had any real eating problems, I became influenced by my colleagues at work and began to eat less and less. All the other girls in the office were on a diet of green salad and apple for lunch. No fats, no meat. Although I didn't notice immediately, my periods had become very irregular. I often missed a month, even two, but I saw this as a bit of a bonus rather than anything to worry about! Then, when it was taking me a long time to become pregnant, my doctor explained that my irregular monthly cycle was making ovulation difficult and that my body was waiting until the 'famine' was over before conceiving a baby. The very next day I began to eat more, but it took a few weeks of forcing myself to eat before I got back my appetite. But all that's ancient history! Now I'm the proud mum of Hugo (three years old) and Laura (two months). »

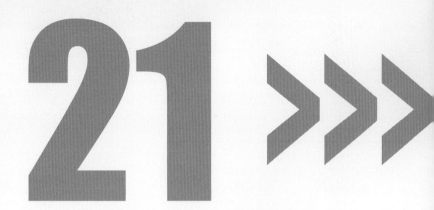

21

»» Yes, of course, it's the mother who produces the baby. But from genetic, biological and biochemical points of view, **the father's role is just as important.** That is why the man is always invited at least to the initial consultation when a couple is finding it difficult to become pregnant.

»»»» **Sperm are produced by men only from puberty onwards,** while the immature eggs are already in a baby girl's ovaries before she is even born.

»»»»» Sperm are therefore particularly affected by their environment, by such factors as diet, toxins and lifestyle. **Many things can disrupt the effectiveness of these minute male sex cells.**

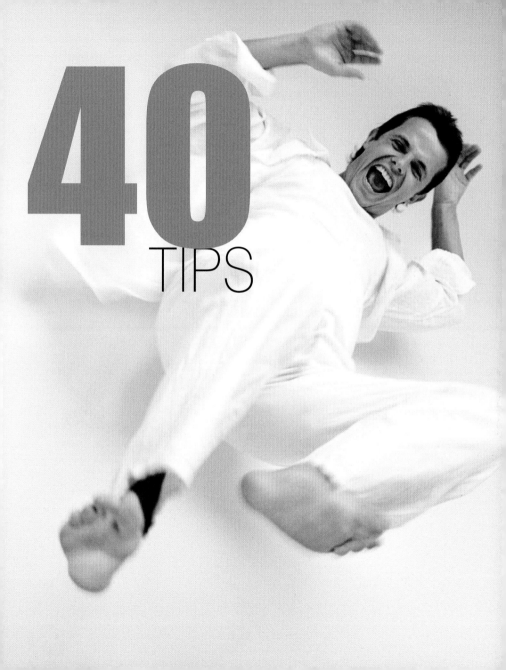

40
TIPS

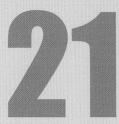

21

three cheers
for your sperm

Don't be too critical of your sperm: put yourself in their place for a moment. These champion athletes have to make enormous efforts to reach their goal. You should applaud their heroism!

It's a cruel world

Competing in the Olympics is a doddle compared with the feats required of sperm once they are in situ. The course they have to cover is fraught with danger, and weak or damaged specimens simply fall by the wayside. Even for the most fit examples, the journey can be compared to taking part in the Tour de France on a bike with flat tyres, using

●●● DID YOU KNOW?

> Sperm are expelled at the remarkable speed of 30kmph (20mph) and then progress through the vagina at 1cm per hour.

> Each one measures 0.07mm long, is a tenth of the thickness of a finger-nail, and weighs a ten-billionth of a gram!

only one leg. Their one aim is to reach the egg: a large, inert cell lying waiting in the body of a woman.

The stress of competition

There are at least 400 million of them on the starting line, but only one winner (or more often than not, no victor at all). Before them lies the crossing of a sticky, thick substance (the cervical mucus), which will stop millions of them in their tracks; a clamber up the uterus; the ascent of a Fallopian tube; and finally a sprint over the last few millimetres to get away from the rest of the pack. And they must do all this while being soaked by secretions, dodging deadly traps and avoiding pitiless sentinels (the white corpuscles). The first to arrive takes the prize, but only if he can penetrate the egg and unite with it.

> Each of these featherweights has a tail, which propels the sperm towards the egg, and even contains a tiny explosive charge to help penetrate the egg membrane.

KEY FACTS

* You should think of your sperm as heroes!

* They have to be extremely fit to accomplish their mission.

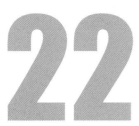

22

When it comes to reproduction, weight problems are much more significant for the woman than the man. However, being either obese or severely underweight can cause him difficulties, too.

climb on the scales

Losing weight or putting it on

Obese men, of course, should attempt to lose weight for the sake of their general health, but, more specifically, obesity can reduce the production of testosterone and cause a loss of libido. Being severely underweight, on the other hand, can lead to a reduction in both the quantity and the quality of the sperm. It is therefore just as important for men as for women to try to eat a

● ● ● D I D   Y O U   K N O W ?

> Gaining weight when you are naturally skinny is quite an art. Above all, don't stuff yourself with junk food all day long: you won't have any appetite left for good, nutritious food.

> Eat more, but choose food that benefits your health and your fertility: some starchy food at every meal (bread, potatoes, pasta, semolina,

balanced diet and to aim for a normal weight if they are thinking of starting a family.

A little exercise

Physical activity is vital both for losing fat (and therefore kilos) and for building muscles (and so gaining weight). What's more, you'll need to be fit once the baby has arrived! The prospect of becoming a father often motivates men with too much flab to finally get rid of some of it. Skinny, underweight men, meanwhile, should seriously think about building up their strength.

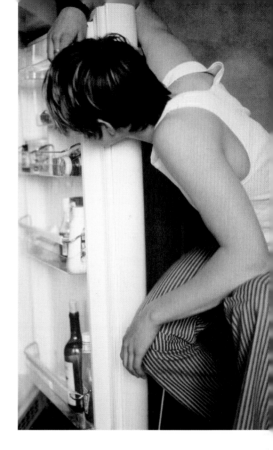

rice, sweetcorn, pulses, chestnuts, lentils, plantains); some red meat and chicken; oily fish (salmon, sardines) as often as possible; a little olive oil.

KEY FACTS

* It's never good to be very overweight or very underweight.

* Choose what you eat carefully, even when you are trying to put on weight.

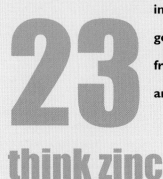

23

think zinc

Zinc is vital for sexual activity. It is involved in the development and functioning of the genital organs. Without it, you would suffer from impotence, absence of sexual pleasure and infertility.

Indispensable for men

Zinc plays a really important role in male fertility. When there's a shortage of it, everything starts to work poorly: the metabolism of testosterone, the production of sperm and even the development of the testicles are all affected. If you increase your intake of food containing zinc, your sperm will become stronger, more numerous and more mobile. As you get older, zinc will also help prevent prostate problems, an area that produces many health difficulties in older men. It's very much a man's mineral.

Precious, but easily lost

It takes a surprisingly long time – some three months – to produce a sperm, and zinc is needed throughout the entire procedure. Not only that, but men lose a little zinc every time they ejaculate, as well as when they urinate and sweat. Some specialists believe that zinc deficiency is one of the major causes of male infertility.

> The best sources of zinc are shellfish, liver and other forms of meat, fish, egg yolk, brewer's yeast, wholegrain cereals and pulses.

KEY FACTS

* Zinc is a key mineral where male fertility is concerned.

* A lack of zinc can be a contributing factor in male infertility.

24 eat more fruit!

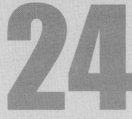

Vitamin C gives sperm a boost, and much more besides. So men who are worried about their fertility would be well advised to give up chocolate mousse and ice-cream and switch to fresh fruit for dessert.

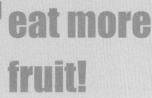

Vitamin C makes everything work better

Vitamin C has often been called the 'anti-tiredness' vitamin, but it has many other beneficial effects. Above all, it's one of the principal antioxidants, which protect the body against the damaging effects of free radicals. Fertility, like everything else, is affected by how well we defend ourselves against these unstable molecules. There's no doubt that everything works better with a good supply of vitamin C. Studies have shown that when the intake of vitamin C is insufficient, the sperm level suffers. Under normal circumstances, the seminal fluid of the testicles contains six to seven times more vitamin C than the blood. In other words, a shortage will reduce the quality of the sperm. This is particularly true if you smoke, as this exacerbates any vitamin C deficiency. Taking a general vitamin supplement is therefore recommended for smokers (although giving up smoking would be an even better idea, of course).

Beware of too much of a good thing

Some specialists also prescribe vitamin C supplements for forms of male infertility due to excessive agglutination (clumping) of the sperm. And there are many other circumstances in which taking vitamin C supplements might be advisable: for example, if you are repeatedly falling ill with infections, if you exercise intensively or if you live in a heavily polluted environment. However, recent research has suggested that taking excessive amounts of vitamin C can cause more harm than good. So only take the high-dosage vitamin C supplements after consulting your doctor.

KEY FACTS

* Vitamin C helps to reduce the damaging oxidation of the body's cells (see Tip 37).

* Try natural supplements such as acerola cherry and rosehip, but consult your doctor before taking high-dosage supplements.

discarding the water is a classic way of ridding food of its vitamin C.

> The body finds it difficult to store, so eat sources of vitamin C on a regular basis.

25 take care if you get on you bike!

Too much mountain biking without taking the necessary precautions can damage the testicles. You need to use the right equipment if you take part in this sport.

Knocks and vibrations: Men who do a lot of mountain biking (5000km/3000 miles per year) are very likely to damage their scrotum. The knocks and vibrations experienced by mountain bikers mean that **88** per cent of them suffer cysts and damaged veins in the scrotal sac, which protects the fragile testes. This compares with just **26** per cent of non-cyclists. What's more, the sperm of cyclists is often of an inferior quality. (They have a low sperm level.)

A few precautions: If you are a cycling enthusiast, protect your scrotum as much as possible. Suitable clothing (padded cycling shorts), a good suspension system and a gel saddle will soften impact. But try, as far as possible, to avoid all impact: raise yourself slightly out of the saddle when negotiating pot-holes and bumps and don't take any unnecessary risks. In fact, do all you can to protect this very delicate and important part of your anatomy.

● ● ● D I D   Y O U   K N O W ?

> The testicles are particularly sensitive to knocks, vibrations, changes in temperature and rubbing.
> If you take part in dangerous sports, such as boxing and wrestling, use all the necessary protective equipment.

KEY FACTS

* Mountain biking can damage the scrotum.

* Make sure you have all the necessary protective equipment.

26 don't forget about selenium

A shortage of the imporatant mineral selenium could lead to feeble and rather lazy sperm!

The key to being a good swimmer: Without selenium, the sperm will not have the energy to stay the arduous course in the vagina. This mineral also helps to promote fertility, particularly male fertility, in plenty of other ways, too: it is utilized in the production of testosterone and is a component of keratin, a vital protein that is found in every sperm's tail.

A versatile mineral: In addition to all of this, selenium is one of the most powerful antioxidants, effectively protecting the reproductive organs against free radicals. It also combats cardiovascular diseases and cancers. Obviously, it is a good idea to include selenium-rich foodstuffs in your diet, and additional supplements can be advisable in certain cases of deficiency.

● ● ● DID YOU KNOW?

> Selenium is a formidable detoxifier, which traps heavy metals (see Tip 32) and removes them from the body. Goodbye lead, cadmium and mercury!

> Our diet doesn't always provide us with sufficient selenium, because the soil in which our crops are grown is not rich in it. The best sources of the mineral are eggs, meat, fish, cereals, lentils, bread and nuts.

KEY FACTS

∗ Selenium promotes fertility, particularly male fertility.

∗ This important mineral can be found in proteins.

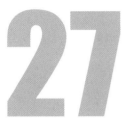**27**

accept that you aren't perfect

It's not all about having sex. There's more to making a baby than simply making love to your partner: your sperm need to be strong, and there needs to be enough of them in the semen.

It's a dual responsibility

In most couples, the woman is usually the first to be 'suspected' of being infertile. For a long time, women were made to undergo a series of unpleasant examinations before it was even considered that it might be their partner who had a problem. Even nowadays, a woman frequently has to have a laparoscopy under general anaesthetic, while her partner merely has to undergo a simple sperm count.

● ● ● DID YOU KNOW?

> Male infertility has only recently (in the 1970s) been 'discovered'.

> This means that much more is known about the female side of the infertility equation than the male, even though it's much easier to collect sperm to study than eggs.

> If conception is proving extremely problematic (trying without success for over two years) it is often both partners that are suffering from low fertility.

'Never tell a man he's infertile'

No, it's not the title of a West End farce. It comes from an endocrinology manual studied by students in the eighties. And not the 1880s; the 1980s! This type of 'advice' is no longer given to medical students, but there remains a prevailing attitude in the medical profession that the male ego must be protected at all costs where fertility issues are concerned. This, of course, can be very counter-productive for couples having trouble conceiving a child. If doctors only look for female problems, those are the only problems they are likely to find. But there is substantial evidence that the semen of many men nowadays is not very fertile. We should at least be more open to the possibility that in cases of difficulty in conceiving, the cause could lie with the male partner, although neither partner should be deemed to be 'at fault'

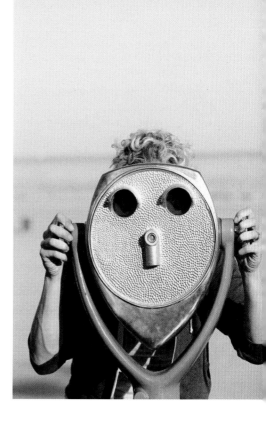

KEY FACTS

* In a significant number of cases, infertility is due to the man.

* If conception is proving very difficult, often both partners are suffering from low fertility.

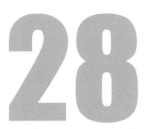

28
look after your blood vessels

The delicate blood vessels that carry blood to the testicles must be 'clean' and not affected by cholesterol or other saturated substances. Otherwise, there may be hardening of the arteries and a poor blood supply to the testicles.

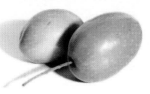

Ensure your circulation is good

The proper functioning of the male genital organs depends on good blood circulation. Sophisticated mechanisms enable the penis to grow erect and the testicles to produce semen. This is why it's of vital importance for the blood to flow freely and the blood vessels to be unobstructed. To achieve this, as with so many things, good diet is essential.

● ● ● DID YOU KNOW?

> Our blood circulation depends largely upon our diet and lifestyle.
> If you eat unwisely, patches of fat develop on the artery walls.

> High blood pressure further complicates this problem, as does diabetes.

Try a Mediterranean diet

It's a fallacy to think that the famous Mediterranean diet is only for octogenarians or victims of coronary heart diesease. In fact, it's quite the opposite. Healthy eating habits will help prevent all illnesses, particularly cardiovascular ones. You need to eat more fruit and vegetables and limit your intake of meat and other animal products (such as butter and cheese), without cutting them out completely. You should also consume plenty of olive oil, nuts and garlic (but make sure your partner eats garlic too if you are trying for a baby!).

> The 'prescription' for both conditions is as follows: reduce your intake of fats (especially saturated and hydrogenated fats), drink less alcohol, don't smoke (it hardens the arteries) and do some physical exercise every day.

KEY FACTS

* Good blood circulation is needed for sexual organs to work properly.

* The Mediterranean diet is good for everybody.

29

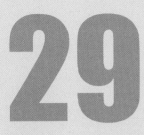

Don't take up yoga just because it's all the rage. Its ancient techniques and teaching can be very beneficial, bringing suppleness to the body and peace to the mind.

the value of yoga

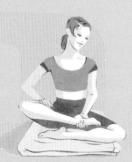

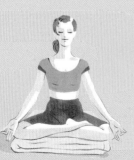

The art of meditation

If your mind tends to wander and you find it hard to concentrate on the task in hand, yoga can help. Use this 6000-year-old discipline to help you relax and meditate on the prospect of having a child. Some people place great faith in the power of thought. Simple meditation and visualization techniques could be beneficial, if only for the purpose of de-stressing.

Siddhasana (perfect posture)

Masters of yoga are able to meditate in any position at any time, but the *Siddhasana* posture provides the novice with an ideal way to concentrate, to forget the body and focus entirely on the subject of meditation.

① Sit on a folded blanket. Hold your right foot in your left hand and bend your right leg so your knee is touching the floor. Bring your foot up against the top of your left thigh, with your heel as close as possible to your body. Bend the left knee and bring your toes up to your other thigh. Your knees should be far apart and your back straight. Reverse your leg positioning if it suits you better.

② Stretch your arms and put your hands on your knees. You can, if you wish, place your thumb and index finger together to make the gesture of knowledge (*Jnana mudra*).

● ● ●　DID YOU KNOW?

> As its name indicates, *Sukhasana* (*sukha* = easy, pleasant) is an easy position to maintain, so it is one you can return to when you are discouraged by the difficulty of some other postures.

① Sit with your legs stretched out in front and close together, your back perfectly straight, your chest pushed forward and your shoulders pulled back.

② Cross your legs in front of you, without letting your knees touch the floor. Place your hands on your knees so that the weight of your body is on your buttocks. Ensure that your back stays very straight.

③ To achieve a complete stretch, raise your arms as far as possible above your head before placing your hands, with palms turned upwards, on your knees.

KEY FACTS

∗ Conceiving a child is not something to be done hastily and carelessly.

∗ Yoga can help you to refocus on your wish to conceive.

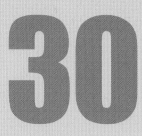

30

boost
your energy!

The change from one season to the next and the stresses of daily life often make us feel listless. You can give yourself an energy boost the Chinese way simply by applying pressure at strategic points with your fingers!

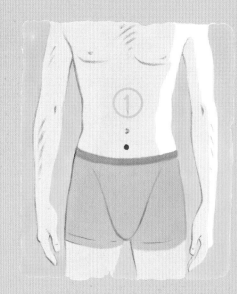

Energy blocks

Chinese medicine is based on the concept that fitness and health depend directly on the way energy circulates in the body. During seasonal changes and times of emotional and physical stress, this energy can be blocked in some of the organs, causing them to be overactive, while other parts of the body are deprived of this vital energy. Each imbalance produces problems, which are often indicated by a loss of energy. If merely getting through the day takes it out of you, how can you hope to father a child?

Little fingers, big effects

To boost energy, acupuncturists place needles in selected parts of the body. You can mimic this treatment by massaging these strategic points with your fingers to help your vital energy circulate correctly. The most accessible points are:

① The navel
An inch or so below the navel.
② The wrist
An inch or so above the point where the wrist bends, between the two bones of the forearm.

③ The knee
The point where the tibia and fibula meet, at the front of the leg, in the hollow under the knee.

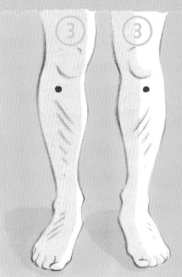

● ● ● DID YOU KNOW?

> When massaging these strategic points, either simply press downwards with your thumb or rub gently using a circular motion.

> Never press so hard that it causes pain, which can easily happen. If your energy is circulating badly, then the treatment points will probably be quite sensitive.

KEY FACTS

* You feel no sense of well-being nor the desire to make love if you have no energy.

* Learn self-massage to help boost your energy.

Many occupational or environmental compounds, including pesticides, solvents and formaldehyde, may affect fertility. They enter our bodies through the skin or respiratory system, affect our immune system and can do a lot of damage.

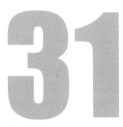

31
avoid glycol
ethers

Infertility, even sterility

Glycol ethers are solvents with many practical uses, but benefiting our bodies isn't one of them. These compounds can harm sperm and intensive exposure could even cause sterility within just a few months. Less frequent contact, such as that which DIY enthusiasts might experience, could double the risk of infertility. These chemicals affect the

● ● ● DID YOU KNOW? ─────────────────────

> There are 80 different glycol ethers.
> The most dangerous belong to the 'e-group' (ethylene). Those in the 'p-group' (propylene) are thought to be less harmful.
> Some ethers have been banned from household products, but others can still be found in glues, shampoos, hair dyes, cosmetic creams, varnish, ink, carpet products, cloths for wiping specta-cles, baby wipes, cleaners, paints, plant-care products... The list goes on and on.

whole process of sperm production and can even prevent them from reaching maturity.

Cancer, too

Some glycol ethers can cause harm to the blood by reducing the number of blood cells and causing anaemia. Others attack the reproductive organs, while some affect the respiratory system. Pregnant women and foetuses are particularly vulnerable, causing damage to the central nervous system and harelips in unborn children. There are also possible carcinogenic effects, especially to the liver and stomach.

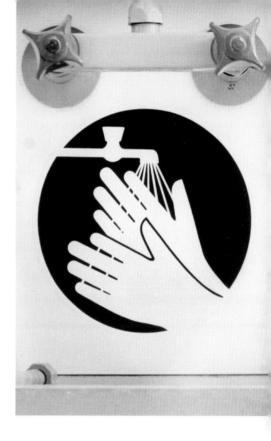

> All DIY products described as being 'water-based' contain some ethers. They are also used intensively in some trades and professions, such as hairdressing, cleaning and maintenance, silkscreen printing, electronics, armaments and even computing.

KEY FACTS

* Avoid all products with 'methyl ethers' or 'ethylglycol' on the label.

* Always open the window when working with chemical products.

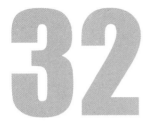

32 beware of heavy metals

Heavy metals are known for the harm they can do to health, including fertility.

A weighty problem: Lead was the first heavy metal to be recognized as harmful to fertility (so significant that it is discussed individually in Tip 39). Cadmium was subsequently also revealed to be toxic for both men and women. However, it can be avoided by giving up smoking (see Tip 41). As for mercury, arsenic, copper, zinc and chrome, none of these causes a problem when absorbed in reasonable quantities, and the last three can be positively beneficial in moderation.

Unfortunately, however, as pollution increases, safe limits are often exceeded.

Under the influence of mercury: We are seldom exposed to mercury, which is fortunate because it is extremely toxic. If, however, you have several fillings in your teeth, the acidity in saliva may cause the mercury in the dental amalgams to escape into your body. If you are concerned by this, you could ask for resin fillings, and avoid eating large fish like tuna, which can be contaminated with mercury. (It should be noted that the British Dental Association states that amalgam fillings are perfectly safe, and it has a great deal of research to support its case.)

●●● DID YOU KNOW? ─────

> Above a certain level, heavy metals become toxic, and they can be harmful even when below this level, if their molecular state is not compatible with human metabolism.
> Environmental pollution can poison us through the food we eat and the air we breathe.

 KEY FACTS

✳ Don't smoke!

✳ Throw away any canned food more than a year old and never store food in opened cans.

33 say it with flowers

Investigating your innermost feelings can be assisted by the use of the right floral elixirs.

A little self-analysis: Floral elixirs can help you overcome your emotional problems. To choose the right remedy you need to carry out a little self-analysis. Ask yourself: am I fearful of something or unsure and discouraged? Do I feel dejected or desperate? Do I feel lonely? Am I too affected by external influences or oddly indifferent to them?

Dr Bach's flower remedies: If you can identify the emotion that's causing your unease, you'll then be able to choose the most suitable flower remedy to treat it. For example, if you are obsessively worried about the pains your wife will experience during childbirth, try taking nutmeg. If you are looking for something to clean out your body, use crab apple. If you are finding it hard to communicate and feel you always want to be alone, try water violet.

● ● ● DID YOU KNOW?

> During the 1930s Dr Bach found that flowers could be effective 'medicines for the emotions'.

> Floral elixirs are totally safe. You can treat yourself without consulting a specialist and can experiment with combinations of several flowers. Just take four drops of tincture (flower essence dissolved in alcohol) three times a day until you feel better.

> If you would rather avoid alcohol, you can dilute the flowers in water.

KEY FACTS

* Negative emotions can have a harmful effect on fertility.

* Floral elixirs can help to calm disturbing emotions.

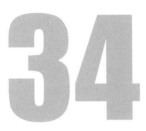

34

hormonal pollution

Some pesticides, plastics and cosmetics interfere with our hormonal system. They contain what are known as 'hormone impostors' or 'endocrine disrupters'. They can affect men by causing a dramatic reduction in the number of sperm produced.

'Hormone imposters'

One of the major causes of the recent reduction in male fertility is exposure to hormones that are increasingly present in the environment. These 'hormone impostors' take the place of our own natural hormones, thereby preventing the latter from carrying out their functions. Among the consequences of this phenomenon are a dramatic increase in hormonal cancer (breast, prostate, testicular) and a worrying decline in the quality of human semen. These synthetic hormones can accumulate in the body (particularly in body fat) and cause long-term damage.

Beware of plastics

Of course, it's difficult to avoid these 'impostors', because they are found everywhere nowadays. To limit the harm they can do, try to avoid 'phthalates'. These are found in the flexible PVC used in plastic food wrapping (mainly for oil, margarine, milk, butter and meat). Never heat these foods in their wrapping, and don't re-wrap them after they've been fried. Avoid toys that are painted and/or made of varnished plastic, particularly if they are flexible and were on sale before 1999. Throw away your oilcloth table covering and get a cotton table-cloth instead. Manufacturers sometimes boast that they have used adipate substances rather than phthalates, but it's debatable if these are any better.

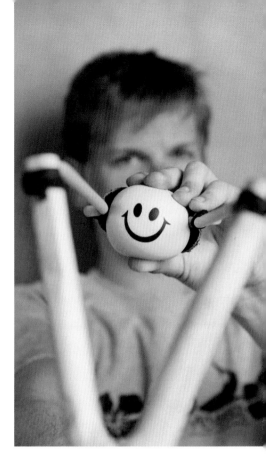

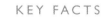 KEY FACTS

* Hormonal pollution is thought to be a major cause of infertility.

* Beware of all types of flexible plastics.

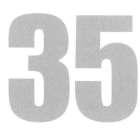

35

briefs or boxers?

This crucial question is far from being resolved definitively. Those who advocate briefs say they provide more support, while those in favour of boxer shorts claim they are sexier. As for the scientists, they are more concerned with temperature control.

Fresh air's the thing!

In nearly 70 per cent of cases of men diagnosed as having fertility problems, the cause is 'unknown'. But this doesn't stop us having our suspicions. One of the most common reasons for ineffective sperm is heat. There's no point moving to Greenland to increase your fertility, however, because it is coolness in the testicular region that is required. Nature's answer to the problem was to

● ● ● DID YOU KNOW?

> If testicles get too hot, a process called molecular acceleration begins within them.

> If, through your job, you are exposed to heat all day long: try to cool down frequently; wear loose, cool, light-coloured clothing; take cool showers (especially in the evening, after work).

design testicles so that they hang just outside the body in the adult male. As a result, doctors tend to advise men to wear boxer shorts to give them some freedom of movement, even if the nether regions are clothed.

Avoid saunas!

And, if briefs aren't healthy, it won't surprise you to learn that saunas should be avoided, too. For the same reasons, sedentary jobs in a hot environment, like cooking or welding, or those that require you to sit down for long periods, like driving, are also likely to damage sperm. Some researchers have even gone so far as to suggest that using disposable nappies on male babies could affect their fertility twenty years down the line. But even if that seems far fetched, the fact remains that testicles need air and coolness.

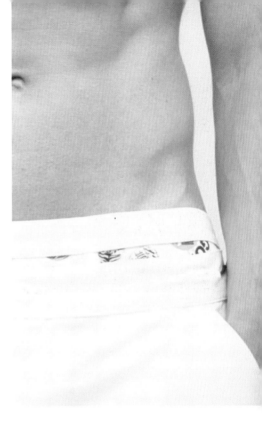

> If you follow these simple rules, the number and mobility of your sperm will quickly return to a satisfactory level.

KEY FACTS

* High temperatures are harmful to sperm.

* Avoid overheated places, long periods of sitting down and saunas.

* Take cool showers.

To stand the best possible chance of improving your fertility, look after your body well. This classic yoga posture induces a deep sense of calm and enables you to get things back into perspective.

36

practice 'the candle'

Head down

In daily life, poor posture can prevent the body's organs from receiving the vital supplies they need. The 'candle' (shoulderstand), like other upside-down stretches, inverts gravity. It enables the muscles and joints to find their correct positions and makes more blood flow to the head, helping you relax and boosting your circulation. The lymphatic system is also stimulated, so cleansing the body. Adopting this position both nourishes the body and helps to eliminate waste. Additional benefits are that the spine is stretched and that the ribcage opens, so improving breathing.

Get down to it!

① Lie down with your feet touching a wall, with your legs bent, so that your hips are as close to the wall as possible. Then put your feet flat against the wall.

② Raise your feet up the wall, without straining. Then bring them down, at the same time lowering your hips onto the floor. Stay in this position for one minute before continuing. Breathe normally.

③ Lie on your back with blankets under the nape of your neck, shoulders and elbows. Keep your head and neck on the floor. Push up from the ground, lifting your hips directly above your head and supporting the small of your back with your palms.

Raise your hips and legs, supporting yourself with your hands pressed against your back. Stretch your chest, hips and legs. Your body should be perfectly straight. Hold the position for five to ten minutes (or until it becomes uncomfortable). To come down, bend your knees while still supporting your back. Place your hands on the ground and return to the starting position.

● ● ● DID YOU KNOW?

> You need to wear loose clothes for this posture and have 15 minutes or so to spare. When you are more used to doing it, you'll find you won't need so much time and will be able to do it easily almost anywhere.

> If you do this exercise regularly, you'll find that you start to eradicate much of the tiredness that accumulates during the day.

KEY FACTS

* Bad posture can prevent some organs in the body from getting the vital supplies they need.

* Don't perform this exercise if you are suffering from an ear infection or high blood pressure.

37 protect yourself from oxidation

Oxidation, caused by free radicals, speeds up ageing and damages the body's organs, including the reproductive system.

● ● ● DID YOU KNOW?

> In some countries, men are encouraged to make an appointment with a doctor before even attempting to start a family. Simple advice on diet, alcohol and avoiding drugs is routinely offered during these consultations.

> Such consultations are not common practice in Britain, but the dietary advice in this book gives men much of the information they will need concerning food and fertility.

Rusty sperm?

Your reproductive cells are extremely vulnerable to attacks by free radicals, so it makes sense to strengthen your antioxidant defences. This is particularly necessary for men, as they produce sperm throughout their adult lives. The testicles do possess an inherent, efficient antioxidant system, but it can be over-whelmed by the assaults of pollutants and stress, or if there is a shortage of antioxidants in the body.

Vitamin C and flavonoids, a winning combination

Aim to eat at least five portions of fresh fruit and vegetables per day, eat simple, healthy food and avoid ready-meals and/or those containing a lot of sugars and fats. Fruit and vegetables are not just for women on diets, as some men seem to think: they are the best sources of vitamin C and flavonoids (such as rutin and quercetin), the most important antioxidants.

KEY FACTS

* Free radicals are proven to harm fertility.

* Eat antioxidant-rich food, such as fresh fruit and vegetables.

> A great deal of research has been carried out into the effects of diet on fertility and the conclusions are indisputable.

38

Urban pollution isn't good for our health, but rural life is not necessarily any better. One study has shown that the sperm of men living in the countryside is of an even poorer quality than that of city dwellers. So much for the rural idyll.

go organic

Pesticides are everywhere

Pesticides are found in parks, at the roadside, in fields, on railway tracks, in gardens, in our houses (wood-treatment products), in our food, flowers, trees, the wind, the clouds, the rain. Although it's difficult to show direct links between chronic exposure to pesticides and health problems, a study conducted in the United States highlighted that farmers in regular contact with these

● ● ● D I D   Y O U   K N O W ?

> Organic agriculture is entirely free of pesticides, environmentally friendly and healthier. We should welcome its increasing success.

> About thirty pesticides have been shown to reduce fertility, cause impotence and endanger pregnancy (miscarriages and birth defects).

chemicals suffer from certain illnesses to a greater extent than the rest of the population. They also have reduced levels of fertility.

Penetrating the water table

More precisely, it seems that the sperm of men exposed to pesticides have significantly reduced mobility and longevity. Some pesticides are considered to be particularly dangerous: DDT, an extensively used pesticide, has been present in soils for a long time now and has soaked into water tables. Some of these products have similar effects to hormonal impostors (see Tip 34), while others are toxic in different ways. As new products are appearing every year and combining with older ones, it is difficult to work out just what the effects on fertility are.

> People frequently in contact with these substances are most at risk, but no one knows the consequences of a daily intake, however small, of pesticides in our food.

KEY FACTS

∗ Eat organic food whenever possible.

∗ If you are a farmer, protect yourself when using pesticides.

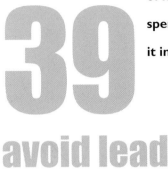

Lead is recognized as a probable cause of male infertility because it damages sperm. But you can take steps to avoid it in your daily life.

avoid lead

A bad sense of direction

Lead can reduce both the number of sperm and their mobility. Researchers have also recently discovered that sperm affected by lead have trouble locating the egg. It is not known exactly how this pollutant upsets their sense of direction, but it seems to damage the receptors that are supposed to guide the sperm.

● ● ● DID YOU KNOW?

> The effect of lead on male fertility is still not fully understood, as it has only recently been identified.

> Lead poisoning known as 'saturnism' or 'plumbism' can affect young children living in houses decorated with lead-based paints.

When the paint deteriorates it gets into household dust and the soil around the house and is easily absorbed by children playing in and around the home.

No one is safe

It's important to note that high levels of lead are not dependent on particular occupations or geographical locations. We are all at risk from it, particularly if our water supply is still fed through lead pipes. It is also found in old paint, the air (petrol fumes) and in workplaces (welding fumes). Of course, air pollution by lead has declined with the advent of lead-free petrol, but soil pollution persists. And scientists have located 133 possible sources of lead poisoning. Tobacco and alcohol both increase the level of lead in the bloodstream. However, foods rich in iron (red meat and eggs) and calcium (dairy products) diminish its absorption. It's also known that physical activity reduces the level of lead in the blood.

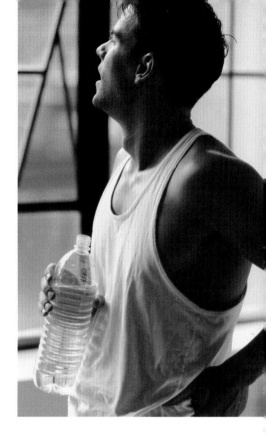

> However, this remains a marginal problem compared with chronic lead poisoning.
> Pregnant women need to be very careful since the foetus, with its rapidly growing brain, is vulnerable to the effects of lead.

KEY FACTS

* If you wish to drink hot water, heat cold water rather than drink hot water directly from the tap.

* You should always let tap water run for a little while before drinking it.

40 Q10 – a useful antioxidant

Well-known as helpful for heart problems, co-enzyme Q10 is also a valiant defender of sperm.

Mobility guaranteed: Free radicals damage the body's organs and cause ageing. Antioxidants reduce, and can even neutralize, their effects. One of them, co-enzyme Q10, plays a significant role in the production of the energy needed by the sperm to maintain their mobility. Co-enzyme Q10 supplements will, therefore, perk up 'tired' sperm.

Getting enough: Your normal food intake should provide you with enough of this substance, but it can easily be destroyed during cooking. It is found in soya beans and their derivatives, such as tofu, and in walnuts, almonds and oils. Spinach contains a lot of it, too, but it needs to be consumed with fat to be easily absorbed. Other sources are oily fish, poultry and other meats.

KEY FACTS

* Co-enzyme Q10 plays an important role in ensuring the mobility of sperm.

* Oily fish, vegetables, soya and beef are good sources of this powerful antioxidant.

case study

« Lydia and I had been trying for a baby without success for two years. After a series of medical examinations, the doctor explained that I had fewer sperm than normal and also that they weren't very mobile. These two factors meant that the situation wasn't very promising. The discussion then turned to my job and, when I told him I was a baker, he asked me if it was hot in the bakery. Well, of course it's hot. He told me heat wasn't good for sperm and advised me to go out as often as possible into the yard and to wear loose-fitting clothes and boxer shorts. I also now try to take several cool showers during the course of the day, and certainly one every morning and evening. Now my sperm level has returned to normal, and, what's more, they seem more energetic. Lydia still isn't expecting, but the doctor says there certainly isn't anything to prevent it happening any more. »

41 »»»

»» **On average, only 7 per cent of couples are unable to conceive a child after three years of trying.** So the odds are in your favour if you plan to start a family. But it's hard to convince yourself of this if you've been trying for months to start a family without success.

»»» **So, each year, thousands of couples consult a doctor because they are starting to worry about their fertility.** And thousands of others become concerned but don't seek medical advice, at least not for the first couple of years.

»»»» Your principal support in this difficult time should be your partner. **If you are having problems conceiving, you must address the issue as a team.**

60
TIPS

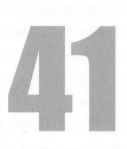

41

no smoking!

Smoking is one of the worst things you can do if you want to conceive. It's certainly very harmful for both men and women, but we may be aware of only the tip of the iceberg in terms of the damage it can do.

When the man smokes

Tobacco is the biggest single cause of male infertility. It lowers the sperm count by between 13 and 17 per cent and has a very damaging effect on the sperm that are produced. In particular, it increases the level of oxidant damage. Nicotine and cadmium, both found in cigarettes, prevent the absorption of the crucial element zinc. Finally, long-term smoking increases erectile dysfunction.

● ● ● DID YOU KNOW?

> Tobacco is highly destructive. It pillages our vitamin reserves, dramatically increasing the amount of vitamins C, B9 and E we need to consume to compensate. All of these vitamins have vital roles to play during pregnancy.

> Smokers often don't have a balanced diet. Their senses of taste and smell are impaired, so they tend to eat foods high in fats and salt.

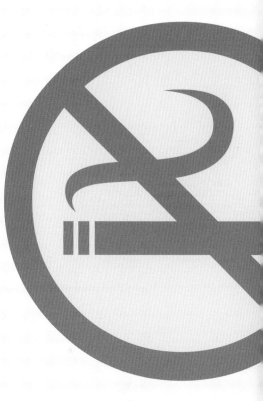

When the woman smokes

Tobacco hampers female fertility by reducing the production of oestrogens. It also increases the risk of ectopic pregnancies, spontaneous abortions and premature births. In addition, it hinders the growth of the foetus and increases the chances of infant death just before, during and just after childbirth. Nicotine narrows blood vessels and causes spasms. As a result, supplies to the placenta are restricted and the foetus is less well nourished.

> At the same time, they find fruit and vegetables less palatable, which exacerbates their vitamin shortages.

42 make love more often

OK, it might seem obvious, but you'd be surprised how many couples become so obsessed by high-fertility periods, temperature curves etc, that they end up not having sex until all the statistics say the time is right. The simplest way to increase your chance of conception is to make love more often.

A question of logic

Some couples find it difficult to conceive a baby for one very simple reason: they make love only once a week. Jobs that involve a lot of travelling, shift work, lack of libido, the demands of other children – there are a thousand and one reasons why modern couples don't make love as often as they might. And if the weekly (or monthly) session doesn't take place when the woman is ovulating, then the prospects are none too bright. Certainly, you shouldn't force yourselves to make love if your heart isn't in it, but it's an undeniable fact that the more you get together between the sheets, the higher will be your chances of success.

Abstinence and fertility

One of the great misconceptions where fertility is concerned, is that if a man abstains for a while, he becomes more fertile. In fact, the opposite is true. Although the number of sperm may increase during 'chaste' periods, they become less mobile and less able to reach the egg. That said, however, several sessions of sexual intercourse each day is also counter-productive, because the man's sperm count is greatly reduced. You need to find a happy medium, which depends on your moods and desire. There are no strict rules.

> But conceiving a child should not become the sole reason for making love. If it is, there'll be a lot of disillusionment down the line.

KEY FACTS

* If your professional lives are out of sync, make a special effort to find times to be together.

* Remember the saying 'eating gives you an appetite'.

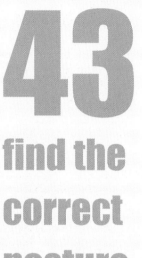

43

find the correct posture

If your body feels stiff, try the Alexander technique. It is based upon the principle that the bad postures we adopt in our daily lives prevent the body from functioning correctly.

The gracefulness of children

The way we move and the postures we adopt habitually every day are often contrary to our bodies' natural stance and movement. This often results in discomfort, tension and pain. Sometimes the pain can be quite severe and noticeable, at others the pain is more of a dull ache, which is easier to ignore. The Alexander technique involves harmonizing body and mind. Children move naturally with

● ● ● DID YOU KNOW?

> At the end of the nineteenth century, the actor Frederick Matthias Alexander noticed that his voice was deteriorating, even disappearing altogether, during performances.

> By observing himself in a mirror, he saw that the muscles in his throat were tensing because he was tilting his head slightly backwards and arching his back, while at the same time stiffening his arms and legs.

much more fluidity and grace than adults, but as we get older the bad habits we develop force the body into repeating movements that interfere with its natural balance.

The turn of a tap

The Alexander technique enables us to learn how to walk, sit down, get up, even turn on a tap correctly. It's all to do with using the minimum amount of effort. For example, when turning on a tap, we waste energy by tensing our neck and back when the movement should just come from the arm. The teacher shows each pupil how to regain natural posture (when resting, walking and so on) and how to be conscious of the way the body feels in order to restore instinctive balance. Good posture and body alignment is obviously important before conception, but it becomes all the more essential during pregnancy.

> From this initial observation has developed a complete system aimed at enabling the body to function better. You'll find the Alexander technique very useful when you are pregnant and trying to avoid uncomfortable positions.

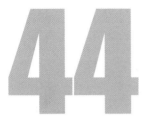

44

seek out
negative ions

Ions are invisible but the air around us is full of them. Unfortunately, there is both a good a bad type. Seek out the negative (the good) to promote good health and reduce anxiety.

What is an ion?

The air is full of oxygen atoms charged with electricity. They are usually 'neutral', but in some circumstances the atoms either lose electrons (and therefore become positive ions) or gain some (becoming negative ions). Contrary to their names, it's the positive ones that make us feel tired and irritable, while the negative ones are both stimulating and relaxing. The kind of ions to which you

● ● ● DID YOU KNOW?

> It's easy to find plenty of negative ions if you're prepared to do a bit of travelling: near waterfalls there are as many as 50,000 per cm³; in the mountains 8000; after a storm 1500 to 2500; in the countryside 500 to 1000. Other sources are: the sun, forests, fountains, waves, a good shower, etc.

> On the other hand, some places swarm with positive ions. This is always the case in confined spaces, such as homes, offices, schools and cars, and anywhere where there is air conditioning.

are exposed depends on your environment: positive ones are found in cities, offices, polluted areas and enclosed places; negative ones in the countryside, in forests, on beaches, in the mountains and close to natural sources of fast-flowing water.

Let ions roam free!

Negative ions are destroyed or damaged by all types of pollutants and air conditioning in enclosed spaces. They are replaced by positive ions, which then proliferate. Among other beneficial biological effects, negative ions stimulate the thyroid gland, the ovaries, the testicles and the secretion of milk, improve alertness, increase alpha waves (relaxation) and reduce anxiety. Positive ions produce exactly the opposite reactions and, in addition, harm sleep patterns and lead to greater aggressiveness.

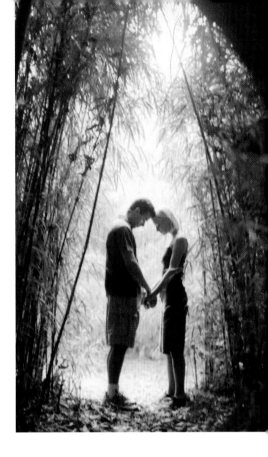

> Other times and situations that produce positive ions are: just before a storm, equinoxes, the full moon, winter, fog, deep valleys, contact with synthetic materials, pollution (tobacco, dust, car fumes) and proximity to electrical equipment, such as televisions and computers.

KEY FACTS

* Get into the countryside as often as possible.

* Buy yourself some plants, opt for coal fires, relax under a long shower.

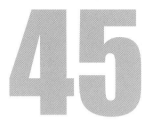

45 take a detox

If your body is full of toxins, heavy metals and other poisons, it's obviously not in the ideal condition to become pregnant.

You need a drink! Many pollutants are harmful to health and interfere with the delicate mechanisms of reproduction. Drinking water is such a simple and everyday thing to do that we often forget about it. However, as soon as we become dehydrated, even slightly, our body suffers and we eliminate waste less efficiently. So drink plenty of water, but choose your water carefully, and look for mineral-rich brands: magnesium 'traps' heavy metals, while calcium protects against lead and cadmium, two pollutants that hinder fertility.

Friendly fibre: Almost everyone should increase their consumption of fibre to help nature's natural process. It benefits the whole body, including the reproductive system. It draws various toxins into the digestive system and then eliminates them from the body in the faeces. It also speeds up bowel movements and so reduces the amount of time pollutants are in contact with the stomach's mucous membranes and it absorbs any free radicals that are lingering in the intestines.

46 you may need to consult a doctor

If you are failing to conceive, the reason may be purely medical, in which case it could also be treatable.

When to suspect a problem: Women may need treatment if they have suffered from menstrual problems, pelvic infections, gynaecological surgery or a complicated case of appendicitis or endometriosis. Men should see a doctor if they have suffered from a hormonal problem such as hypogonadism (underactivity of the testicles), cryptorchidism (testicles not dropping in early adolescence), inflammation of the testicles, venereal disease, a hernia, a varicocele (swelling of a vein in the spermatic cord), excessive weight gain or pre-diabetes.

Bad sex: The majority of reproductive problems have a psychological, nutritional or sexual cause. The man may be impotent or have premature ejaculations, or the woman may find intercourse painful (dysparunia). Any one or a combination of these problems can lead to infrequent sexual relations, and a reduction in the chances of conception.

KEY FACTS

∗ Some medical causes of infertility need treatment.

∗ See your doctor as soon as you can if you are suffering from an illness.

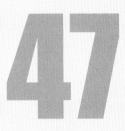

47

cocktails and
pregnancies
don't mix!

'A drink or two can't do any harm.'
Unfortunately, yes it can. This is one
pleasure that it's best to forgo once
you start trying for a baby, and
especially once you have actually
become pregnant.

A glass of water, please

Nothing undermines the male libido as
much as alcohol, because it reduces the
level of testosterone, the key male
hormone. Everyone knows that male
alcoholics have erection problems, but
many men still believe that regular, moderate drinking can't do them any harm.
But this raises the question of what,
exactly, is 'moderate' drinking? Guide-
lines vary from country to country, but

an acceptable amount is generally held to be around a pint and a half a day. Nevertheless, some men find this ridiculously conservative, believing they can safely drink much more. However, if you are one of the men who laugh in the face of the medical advice, the chances are that your sperm are not as numerous or as mobile as they should be.

No alcohol during pregnancy

It is now widely recognized that women should not drink at all during pregnancy. Regular alcohol consumption at this time can lead to foetal abnormalities and behavioural problems. And consuming alcohol before conception can be almost as harmful. If there is alcohol in your system as the sperm reaches the egg and when the delicate process of cell division begins, long-term damage could be the result.

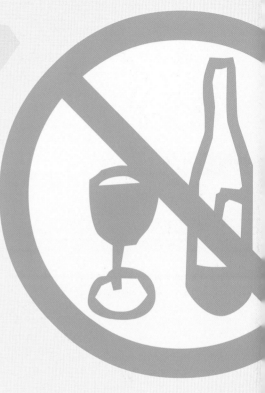

> This umbrella term encompasses a number of conditions, including impaired growth, skull or face deformities, behavioural problems, attention deficit disorder and other learning problems, coordination difficulties and even psychoses.

KEY FACTS

* Alcohol affects the fertility of both sexes and the health of the foetus.

* Stop drinking before you try to conceive.

48 don't wait too long

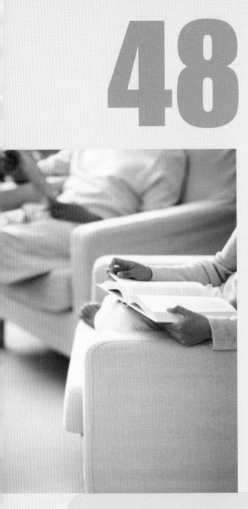

The average age of a first pregnancy is now 28. In 1970 it was 24. Of course, it's good to be able to choose when you want to have children, but be careful not to wait too long.

The most fertile age

Female fertility is at its peak at 25. It then stays on a plateau until 35, when it gradually starts to go into a decline. It falls much more rapidly from around the age of 40. And as the chances of conceiving at all decrease, so the chances of complications during pregnancy rise with age. The same applies to men: their age of maximum fertility is also 25. As they get older, blood supply to the testicles is reduced and the quality of the semen deteriorates. The deterioration in the quality of the semen is due to exposure to pollution and to common illnesses, such as diabetes, which also causes erectile difficulties.

sterility'. So, while it is a fact that fertility generally declines after 35, it's counterproductive to let this worry you. And, as with all health issues, a woman's period of fertility varies enormously from individual to individual. Thousands of women have enjoyed wholly uncomplicated first pregnancies over the age of 35. Many 42-year-olds are still eminently fertile. The most important thing is that the new baby should experience the best possible start in life in an environment of trust, love and, if possible, material stability.

'Stress sterility'

Fear of the 'biological clock' traumatizes many women, and some psychologists believe that this contributes to 'stress

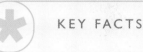

KEY FACTS

* You are generally less likely to become pregnant as you get older.

* However, better a late child than an unwanted one.

> The same applies to men. A 40-year-old non-smoker might well have a better chance of fathering a child than a 25-year-old who smokes 60 a day.

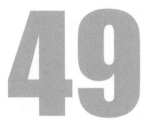

As everyone knows, exercise is good for your health – but not always in the way you might expect. Ladies, if sweating on an exercise mat doesn't turn you on, try sneaking into the men's changing rooms!

the power of pheromones!

Exercise, the great hormonal regulator

It's simple: everything works better if you exercise, especially ovulation. Women who exercise feel fitter, are healthier and suffer fewer hormonal imbalances. Exercise also makes it more likely that you'll have a balanced diet, while reducing stress and improving sleep. None of this is news, of course. But we have learnt recently that the female partners of sportsmen themselves benefit from their man's physical activity. That changing-room smell is more potent than you realized!

Two in one

Recent research has revealed that men's perspiration has a dual effect on women: the smell both improves their mood and boosts their hormonal secretions. Pheromones, hormonal secretions, are the magic ingredients in male sweat. The level of female LH (luteinizing hormone), which triggers ovulation when produced in sufficient quantities, rises when women smell their sweaty partners.

> This phenomenon is not exclusive to humans: our sweat contains the same chemical substance, 5-alpha-androsterone, as a pig's. When emitted by the male, the sow automatically assumes the coupling position.

KEY FACTS

* Exercise is good for hormones and therefore good for fertility.

* The smell of male perspiration can cause women to ovulate earlier than normal.

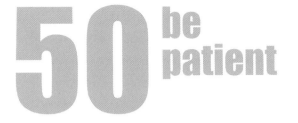

50 be patient

Doctors always remind couples wanting to start a family that they must be patient.

A five-to-one shot: To make a baby, you need a man, a woman, passion and some luck. On average, it takes five to six months for all the right conditions to coincide (a good level of fertility in both partners, the right moment in the menstrual cycle, absence of stress and so on) so that the happy event can occur. Doctors estimate that the success rate is about 20 per cent. In other words, every time you have unprotected sex, there's a five-to-one chance that you'll make a baby. That's why there's little point in seeing a doctor until you have been trying unsuccessfully for at least a year. The doctor will probably simply tell you that you've been 'unlucky' so far.

20 million copies: If 20 million sperm crowd into each millilitre of semen, and they are energetic, good swimmers, the man's fertility is considered 'normal'. If there are only 5 million, then his sperm count is deemed low and the conventional odds of five to one will lengthen accordingly. As a result, conception is likely to take longer, but you should remember that you can beat even high odds if you try for long enough.

● ● ● DID YOU KNOW?

> Although the 'ideal' age as far as fertility goes is 25, many women have given birth to healthy babies well into their forties, and men have been known to father children at the age of ninety!

> Such statistics indicate that it's (almost) never too late to give up hope.

KEY FACTS

∗ It's important to remember that you can increase your chances of conception through perseverance.

∗ No two couples are alike.

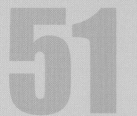

51 springtime: the season of love

A woman is most likely to become pregnant in the spring. Well, that's the theory, anyway.

The season of fertility: Chinese tradition has it that in spring the spirits of the sky and earth are reunited. And a serious scientific study has also found that spring is the ideal time to conceive. Everything seems more set fair at this time: for instance, the chances of successful conception (including through in vitro fertilization) are greater and the embryos tend to be healthier.

The rhythms of the seasons: Nature can sometimes seem strange. For example, female hormonal rhythms are exactly the opposite of male ones. Feminine sexual neurohormones, which originate in the pituitary gland, are produced in great quantities between January and June, peaking in March. Once they are in decline, men's hormones start to increase, reaching a height from June to December. The male sexual urge therefore peaks in August, a good four months after women.

KEY FACTS

* Spring appears to be the best season for making love.

* Redouble your efforts at this time and you might well be rewarded.

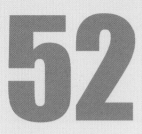

52

do you really want a baby?

Some women are convinced that they want a child while not being at all certain that they can cope with pregnancy and birth. In these circumstances, when stress and uncertainty take their toll psychologically, failure to conceive is likely to continue.

It's all in the mind

Some women claim with absolute certainty that they want a baby, but when they talk to a psychologist, they express widely held fears that reveal serious doubts. Is he really the right man to be the father of my child? Will I be able to look after the infant? Do I really want a baby or do I just want to be pregnant? Do I want a baby just because my friends are having babies? Is my mother pushing me into this pregnancy because she wants a grandchild? It's completely natural to ask yourself such questions, provided you don't become obsessed by them. Talking to a psychologist sometimes throws light on possibly irrational worries or enables you to find the answer to an apparently insoluble conundrum.

Don't block out your child!

It's difficult to estimate how many cases of infertility are caused by such psychological barriers, but increasingly it seems to be a significant number. Certainly, before starting a course of ART, you should fully discuss your situation with a trained psychologist. One of the clearest examples of how emotions may affect fertility can be found in the way some women stop menstruating when they are under extreme stress.

KEY FACTS

* What's going on in your head affects your fertility.

* A psychologist can help you to understand your attitude to having a baby.

Ginger is supposed to be an aphrodisiac, so why not try it if your libido needs a bit of a boost?

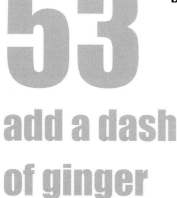

53

add a dash of ginger spice

A versatile plant

Ginger root isn't a love potion, and it won't solve all of your relationship problems, but it could provide a little help when you are feeling tired and romance seems crushed by those day-to-day preoccupations. The magic, such as it is, is held in ginger's oil: simultaneously peppery and lemony, it's very hot, and hopefully will make you feel that way, too! Furthermore, it has undeniable

● ● ● DID YOU KNOW?

> For 'fruit salad for lovers', you need 100g (4oz) each of peaches, strawberries, melon, grapefruit and nectarines; 50g (2oz) of grated ginger; 50g (2oz) of maple syrup or honey; and 500ml (1 pint) of water.

> Bring the water to the boil and then add the maple syrup (or honey). Drop in the grated ginger. Then allow the mixture to cool completely.

medicinal qualities: ginger calms tension, stimulates the senses and is great for relieving nausea, tiredness and chills.

The root with a thousand good qualities

Although its taste is very strong, ginger can be used in numerous dishes, both savoury and sweet. And its spicy, intoxi-cating fragrance is not found only in the kitchen. When it is added to perfumed candles, soaps or shampoos, this aroma can set the bathroom alight! Ginger scented perfume and eau de toilette, often combined with the cooler qualities of citrus fruits, aniseed or flowers, could seduce you for an evening … or even a lifetime.

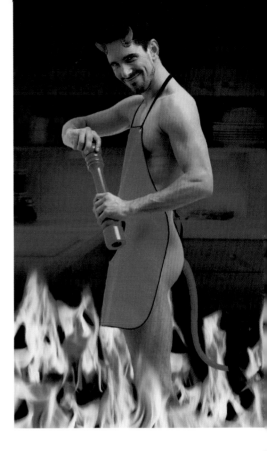

> Cut up the fruit and pour the syrup over it. Put everything in the refrigerator for two hours. Serve with finger biscuits.

KEY FACTS

* Ginger is widely believed to be a natural aphrodisiac.

* Don't expect miracles, but it does contain genuine active ingredients.

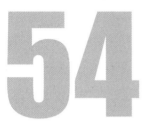

54

clean up your act!

Certain jobs are particularly likely to expose people to toxic substances harmful to their fertility. Although changing jobs is often not an option, there are precautionary measures you can take to try to protect yourself.

Dangerous toxins

The children of firefighters are more likely than other children to suffer from deformities. This is because firefighters often breathe in toxins produced by burning plastics, carpets, and so on. These toxins can seriously damage the firefighters' sperm. Heavy smokers suffer from the same kind of poisoning, as do factory workers (particularly those who work with solvents or rubber), hair-dressers, cleaners (cleaning products), painters and decorators.

Taken to the cleaner's

Female dry cleaners breathe in per-chlorethylene every day and run twice the risk of suffering a miscarriage than other mothers-to-be. We can't all escape pollutants by going to live on a farm in the depths of the countryside, but remember that sensitivity to them is increased if we don't eat enough protective nutrients (especially magnesium and antioxidants such as vitamins C and E, beta-carotene and polyphenols). Don't forget the dangers caused by drinking too much alcohol, which can affect the sperm quality and the foetus.

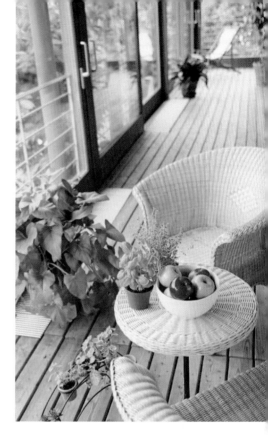

> Don't forget to keep the air circulating inside your house, and keep plants that purify the atmosphere, such as the fig, ivy and dieffenbachia, in your rooms.

KEY FACTS

* Air your rooms regularly.

* Try to increase your intake of antioxidants.

* Buy yourself some plants that help purify the air.

55

that gentle touch...

If you or your partner don't feel particularly well, and you don't know what to do about it, why not try microkinesitherapy? This alternative therapy aims to remove the blockages responsible for infertility.

Putting a smile back on your face

If you're continually plagued by tendinitis, suffering from pains that just won't go away or have a health problem that drags on and on, the answer might be a session of microkinesitherapy. The therapist could also help you if you have a fertility problem, provided the doctors haven't found anything organically wrong with you. This is a very gentle, precise technique that can be effective after just one session and release you from a trauma that might have occurred a long time in the past and damaged your body particularly badly.

Let your body speak

During a microkinesitherapy session, you lie down (fully clothed), while the fingers of the therapist gently touch you, sometimes seeming merely to brush across your clothes, sometimes massaging you gently. The fingers are 'listening' to what your body has to say. The therapist is searching for hidden problems or weaknesses that may have their root cause in an incident that occurred long ago.

> Practitioners seek to relieve blockages that might have occurred long ago, and eradicate their physical symptoms: muscular, skeletal and abdominal pains, headaches and even infertility.

KEY FACTS

* Microkinesitherapy could be termed a kind of psychoanalysis of the body.

* For additional alternative therapies, see Tip 15.

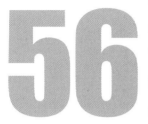

56

get a good night's sleep

Make love as much as you want. Party, in moderation. But always leave yourself enough time to get all the sleep you need. This is a precious time for the body while it regenerates itself in order to be on top form during the day.

Bad sleep, bad mood

The body needs sleep to repair itself, to renew cells, to produce certain hormones, simply to function correctly. If you deprive it, even partially, of this priceless and free source of energy, it soon starts to malfunction. Normally, it's obvious when you are suffering from severe insomnia – you sleep badly and feel tired in the daytime – but it's not

●●● DID YOU KNOW?

> It's vital to eat correctly. Avoid red meat in the evening. Chicken and turkey, on the other hand, contain tryptophane, which aids sleep. This compound is also found in brown rice, bananas, maize and ginger.

> Pasta, potatoes and rice are also good choices for the evening, as they are sleep-inducing.

always as clear cut as that. It's possible to sleep badly without realizing it and wonder why you feel irritable and listless. This happens, for example, if you sleep in a noisy environment or if you have been particularly stressed during the day.

Very active nights

When you are asleep, your body busies itself with some crucial tasks. A tired body inevitably means a grumpy mood, reduced libido and, above all, a lack of efficiency in performing its usual daily functions. Sleep is absolutely essential for health and must be prepared for correctly, from the morning onwards. Eat well during the day so that a few hours before bedtime you can eat just a light dinner that will not interfere with your sleep.

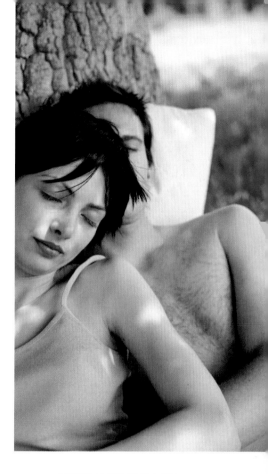

> Oily nuts (almonds, walnuts), pulses (for B vitamins and magnesium) and water with a high mineral content (for calcium and magnesium) are also recommended.

KEY FACTS

* You must get enough sleep.

* Some foods help you to sleep, while others do quite the opposite.

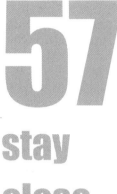

57

stay
close

It would be a pity to allow the desire for a child to threaten your passion for your partner and potentially spoil your relationship.

Make love because you are in love

If you are finding it difficult to conceive, you might start to 'blame' your partner. This is likely to be detrimental to your relationship and will be no help in trying to start a baby. It is easy to allow a vicious circle to develop in which the sole purpose of the relationship becomes the desire for a baby. As a result, sex becomes stressful and less

●●● DID YOU KNOW?

> The desire for a baby is often ambivalent. Of course, it reflects the natural wish to start a family, but many people also think that a baby will cure all the problems in their relationship. This can be a fatal error, which ends in separation.

> Remember that you, your partner and the unborn baby are three distinct entities. Don't count on a baby to improve your relationship. If you are suffering from an undiagnosed case of depression, a baby won't be a cure.

pleasurable and so you feel less like making love, the very thing that you need to do in order to create a baby!

A desire for love

Don't let the situation spiral out of control. You might be depressed, but your partner is almost certainly feeling exactly the same way, and there's no point in making matters worse. The psychologists are categorical: the more you focus on the desire for a child and the more you are afraid of being infertile, the less chance there is of conception, especially if the relationship has hit a rough patch. Some therapists even suggest that the child might not really be wanted at all: the supposed desire for one is, in fact, the expression of a need for love on the part of one or both partners. In such circumstances – and perhaps it is no bad thing – conception often isn't forthcoming.

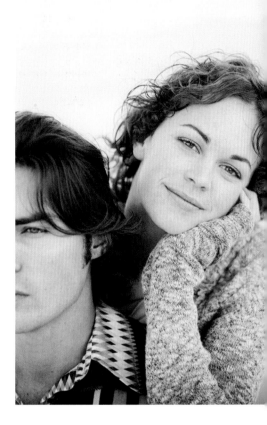

KEY FACTS

* You mustn't jeopardize your relationship if a baby doesn't come.

* Make sure you understand clearly why you want a child.

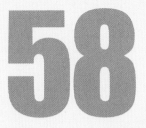

58

nutritional supplements can help

Research shows that nutritional supplements can improve fertility, as well as help protect the mother-to-be and the unborn child.

A perfect world

In an ideal world, supplements would not be needed. Our food would be rich in vitamins and minerals, we would eat perfectly balanced diets, no one would smoke and there would be no pollution. We would all take the correct amount of exercise and nobody would feel stressed. Of course, in reality things are very different, and increasing numbers of doctors are aware that a shortage of micronutrients can cause a huge range of problems, including reduced fertility.

Supplements for your needs

It is true that nearly all of us could improve our diet. But, even if we did, our vitamin intake (particularly B, C and E) would be unlikely to satisfy the body's requirements. Studies show that zinc, folic acid, magnesium or vitamin C sup- plements can help improve the quality of sperm and restore lost libido. Choose supplements according to your needs: vitamin C for smokers (see Tips 24 and 41); folic acid for women (see Tip 9) and men who have certain problems with their semen; other B-group vitamins after having been on the pill (see Tips 10 and 11); iron if you used an IUD (see Tip 19); and zinc to stimulate desire (see Tip 23).

> The nutrients in question are magnesium, zinc, folic acid and vitamin B6. They all work well together, so multi-supplement pills containing them as well as vitamin C and beta-carotene are ideal.

KEY FACTS

∗ Our food intake doesn't always provide us with all the vitamins and minerals we need.

∗ Supplements can sometimes help to restore fertility.

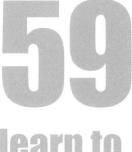

59

learn to relax

Stress is one of the great killers of the modern age. Among many other pernicious effects, it damages our sexual hormones. Avoid it in every way you can, and learn to recognize its many disguises.

Stress and hormones

As everyone knows, stress can trigger a series of physical reactions. For example, when we experience great anxiety, the palms of our hands become clammy and moist. This is an outward sign of a hormonal response to stress. Other hormonal responses are not so visible but just as real. For example, stress disturbs the production of eggs in the ovaries, and every woman knows that experiencing strong emotions can disrupt her periods.

Men are affected, too

Men are not spared from stress or its effects, either. Powerful, painful emotions can result in a reduction in the level of the male hormone testosterone, and/or disrupt the production of sperm. Stress can also eliminate the desire to make love. You might think that it's impossible to relax, given the stresses of your job, your home life, money worries or other anxieties, but there are many things you can do to relieve stress, such as yoga, sport, massage, meditation. It is certainly important to take steps to de-stress your life if you want to start a family.

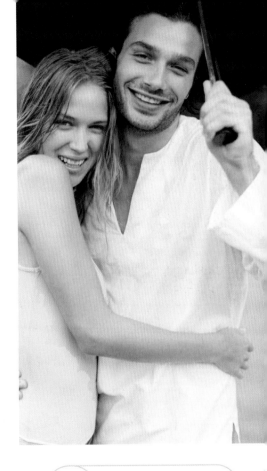

> When the stress is very violent (a shock) or prolonged (a bad atmosphere at home or in the office), the body's capacity to cope with the physical effects is reduced and illnesses can occur.

KEY FACTS

* Working out a relaxation programme is a top priority.

* Rest, walks in the countryside and meditation are all good ways to relax.

60 just say 'no'

Drugs of all kinds, both legal and illegal, and those prescribed by doctors or sold over the counter, can have a profound effect on fertility for men and women.

Cut down on alcohol and cigarettes

Recent research suggests that smoking tobacco drastically affects fertility (see Tip 41). Cannabis should be avoided as much as, if not more than, tobacco. And although moderate alcohol consumption appears to have no detrimental effect on sperm, evidence suggests that excessive drinking dramatically lowers the sperm count (see also Tip 47).

Strong drugs = weak sperm

Anabolic steroids, cocaine and some prescribed drugs can all contribute to reduced male fertility. Opium and its derivatives tend to cause weight loss and, in women, interfere with ovulation. Along with cocaine, they can also seriously harm the foetus, psychologically as well as physically, if taken during pregnancy. It's difficult to determine precisely how much damage such drugs can do, but, certainly the best advice is to avoid them entirely.

●●● DID YOU KNOW?

> It is not only recreational drugs that influence fertility.

> Some drugs that are widely prescribed for medical conditions such as hypertension and depression can affect sexual functioning.

> However, if you're trying for a baby, consult your doctor before you stop taking any prescribed medication.

KEY FACTS

* Alcohol, cigarettes, anabolic steroids and cocaine can all reduce male fertility.

* Other drugs can affect sexual performance in men and ovulation in women.

* Pregnant women should avoid all drugs, including alcohol and caffeine.

case study

We love each other and that's what counts

« We'd been trying for a child for several months with no success. Each of us was sure that the other was the cause of the problem, and we grew irritable and moody with each other. The situation became unbearable, because all we thought about was having a baby. We were making love only during the fertile period of the cycle. The rest of the time we hardly said a word to each other. Things got so bad that we even thought of separating. Paradoxically, that's what brought us back together, because each of us imagined what life would be like without the other and we couldn't bear the thought of it. We ended up deciding that having a baby wasn't so important that we should let it drive us apart; and we didn't opt for IVF treatment because, if our bodies couldn't produce a baby, there was no point in 'forcing' nature. We forgot all about the 'best time of the month' and ovulation tests and went back to the way we had been before without too many regrets. And now we're going to be parents in five months' time! »

useful addresses

» Fertility

Infertility Network UK
Charter House
43 St Leonards Road
Bexhill-on-Sea
East Sussex TN40 1JA
Helpline: 08701 188 088
www.infertilitynetworkuk.com

**International Planned
Parenthood Federation**
Regent's College
Inner Circle
Regent's Park
London NW1 4NS
tel: 0207 487 7900
www.ippf.org

Western Hemisphere
Region:
120 Wall Street
9th Floor
New York
NY 10005
USA
tel: 212 248 6400
www.ippf.org

**International Council
on Infertility Information
Dissemination Inc.**
PO Box 6836
Arlington
VA 22206
USA
tel: 703 379 9178
www.inciid.org

Resolve
7910 Woodmont Avenue
Suite 1350 Bethesda
MD 20814
USA
tel: 301 652 8585
www.resolve.org

**The Fertility Society
of Australia**
61 Danks Street
Port Melbourne
Victoria 3207
tel: 9645 6359
www.fsa.au.com

» Specialist organisations

ACeBabes
(for families following
assisted conception)
www.acebabes.co.uk

The Daisy Network
(support group for women
suffering from premature
menopause)
www.daisynetwork.org.uk

**National Endometriosis
Society**
Helpline: 0808 808 2227
www.endo.org.uk

The Miscarriage Association
Helpline: 01924 200799
www.miscarriageassociation.
org.uk

Verity
(self-help organisation for
women with Polycystic
Ovary Syndrome)
www.verity-pcos.org.uk

» Herbal medicine

**British Herbal Medicine
Association**
Sun House, Church Street
Stroud, Gloucester GL5 1JL
tel: 01453 751389

**National Institute
of Medical Herbalists**
56 Longbrook Street
Exeter, Devon EX4 6AH
tel: 01392 426022

» Yoga

The British Wheel of Yoga
25 Jermyn Street
Sleaford
Lincs NG34 7RU
tel: 01529 306 851
www.bwy.org.uk

» Alexander Technique

**The Society of Teachers of
the Alexander Technique**
1st Floor, Linton House
39-51 Highgate Road
London NW5 1RS
0845 230 7828
www.stat.org.uk

index

acknowledgements

Cover: T. Grill/Iconica; p. 8-9: A.Green/Zefa; p.15: H.Scheibe/Zefa; p.19: A. Normandin/Masterfile; p.21: Grace/Zefa; p.23: R.Holz/Zefa; p.24: R. Minsart/Masterfile; p.27: N. Hendrickson/Masterfile; p.31: M. Alberstat/Masterfile; p.38: J. Burrell/Masterfile; p.41: M. Alberstat/Masterfile; p.45: K. Finlay/Masterfile; p.48-49: K. Murray/Getty Images; p.51: J. Feingersh/Masterfile; p.53: M.Moellenberg/Zefa; p.55: Creaps/Getty Images; p.56: M. Alberstat/Masterfile; p.61: N. Hendrickson/Masterfile; p.63: B. Hagiwara/Getty Images; p.69: J.Westrich/Zefa; p.73: S. Craft/Masterfile; p.75: Star/Zefa; p.78: N. Hendrickson/Masterfile; p.81: Mika/Zefa; p.83: P. Arsenault/Masterfile; p.86-87: A.Green/Zefa; p.90: A. J. Pho/Photonica; p.93: A. Olney/Masterfile; p.95: D. Roth/Getty Images; p.100: R. Febling/Masterfile; p.103: Creasource/Zefa; p.107: J. Pumfrey/Getty Images; p.109: U.Krejci/Zefa; p.111: Neo Vision/Photonica; p.113: P. Boorman/Getty Images; p.115: P.Berry/Zefa; p.117: J. Tisne/Geety Images; p.119: J. Toy/Getty Images; p.121: S.Krouglikoff/Zefa

Illustrations: Anne Cinquanta: p 64-65, 66-67, 76-77

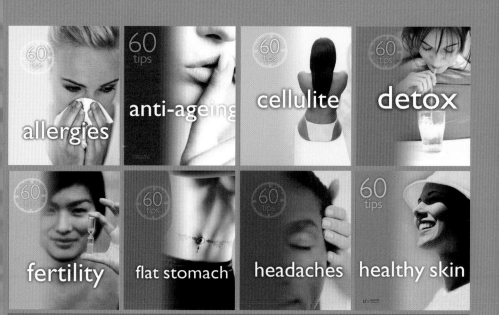

allergies

anti-ageing

cellulite

detox

fertility

flat stomach

headaches

healthy skin

The 60 Tips collection

All the keys, all the tips and all the answers

to your health questions

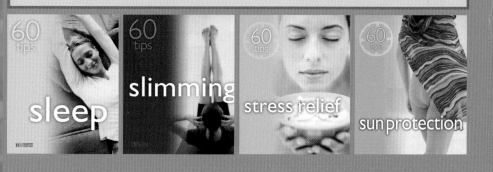

sleep

slimming

stress relief

sun protection

Series editor: Marie Borrel

Director : Stephen Bateman

Editorial director: Pierre-Jean Furet

Editor: Caroline Rolland

Editorial assistant: Maryem Taje

Graphic design and layout: G & C MOI

Copy preparation: Marie-Claire Seewald

Final checking: Dominique Montembault

Illustrations: Guylaine Moi

Production: Caroline Artémon

Translation: JMS Books LLP

© Hachette Livre (Hachette Pratique) 2004
This edition published by Hachette Illustrated UK, Octopus Publishing Group Ltd.,
2–4 Heron Quays, London E14 4JP

English translation by JMS Books LLP (email: Janem030@aol.com)
Translation © Octopus Publishing Group Ltd. 2005

A CIP catalogue for this book is available from the British Library

ISBN 10: 1-84430-136-2

ISBN 13: 978-1-84430-136-2

Printed by Toppan Printing Co., (HK) Ltd.